Advance praise for *Proof of Heaven*

"If Central Casting was given an assignment to locate the most highly qualified person who has had a near-death experience (NDE) to have him write a book about it, lecture about it, and appear in the media to promote it around the world, no one could find a more perfect candidate than neurosurgeon Eben Alexander III, M.D. He has all the necessary academic credentials for this assignment, is warm emotionally, very articulate, has undergone a profound spiritual transformation, and is highly motivated to unify science with spirituality." —Bill Guggenheim, coauthor of *Hello From Heaven!*

"Dr. Alexander's neuroscience career taught him that near-death experiences are brain-based illusions, and yet his personal experience left him dumbstruck. His honest struggle to make sense of this unforgettable journey is a gripping story, unique in the literature of spiritual experiences, that may well change how we understand our role in the universe." —Bruce Greyson, M.D., co-editor of *The Handbook of Near-Death Experiences*

"[T]his important book . . . has the potential to break many scientific taboos." —Pim van Lommel, M.D., author of *Consciousness Beyond Life*

"Eben Alexander brings a unique perspective to the sacred world combining a glorious, personal vision of spiritual consciousness with patient, insightful scientific inquiry. *Proof of Heaven* is a compelling story of what may lie ahead for all of us in the life beyond this one. We have nothing to fear." —Allan J. Hamilton, M.D., author of *The Scalpel and the Soul*

"Dr. Eben Alexander's story of his near-death experience is astonishing. . . . His brushes with the Sublime are exhilarating to read." —Rabbi Neal Gold, Temple Shir Tikva

"Dr. Alexander's experiences resonate remarkably with views of Heaven, the Afterlife, and the potential of consciousness in the Jewish mystical tradition. This book is a thunderbolt!" —Dr. Rabbi Meir Sendor

"Eben's masterpiece is a story for scientists, skeptics, believers, and seekers. Read it for a foretaste of something beyond the veil, beyond our dreams, and beyond our wildest imaginations." —The Rev. Michael R. Sullivan, Rector, Holy Innocents' Episcopal Church, Atlanta, GA

PROOF

of

HEAVEN

A Neurosurgeon's
Journey into the Afterlife

Eben Alexander, M.D.

SIMON & SCHUSTER PAPERBACKS
New York   London   Toronto   Sydney   New Delhi

> *This book is dedicated to all of my loving family,*
> *with boundless gratitude.*

Simon & Schuster Paperbacks
A Division of Simon & Schuster, Inc.
1230 Avenue of the Americas
New York, NY 10020

First Simon & Schuster trade paperback edition October 2012

SIMON & SCHUSTER PAPERBACKS and colophon are registered trademarks of Simon & Schuster, Inc.

The names of some individuals in this book have been changed.

For information about special discounts for bulk purchases, please contact Simon & Schuster Special Sales at 1-866-506-1949 or business@simonandschuster.com.

The Simon & Schuster Speakers Bureau can bring authors to your live event. For more information or to book an event, contact the Simon & Schuster Speakers Bureau at 1-866-248-3049 or visit our website at www.simonspeakers.com.

Designed by Renata Di Biase

Manufactured in the United States of America

29   30

Library of Congress Cataloging-in-Publication Data is available.

ISBN 978-1-4516-9518-2
ISBN 978-1-4516-9519-9 (pbk)
ISBN 978-1-4516-9520-5 (ebook)

Contents

PROOF

of

HEAVEN

PROLOGUE

A man should look for what is,
and not for what he thinks should be.

—ALBERT EINSTEIN (1879–1955)

When I was a kid, I would often dream of flying. Most of the time I'd be standing out in my yard at night, looking up at the stars, when out of the blue I'd start floating upward. The first few inches happened automatically. But soon I'd notice that the higher I got, the more my progress depended on me—on what *I* did. If I got too excited, too swept away by the experience, I would plummet back to the ground ... hard. But if I played it cool, took it all in stride, then off I would go, faster and faster, up into the starry sky.

Maybe those dreams were part of the reason why, as I got older, I fell in love with airplanes and rockets—with anything that might get me back up there in the world above this one. When our family flew, my face was pressed flat to the plane's window from takeoff to landing. In the summer of 1968, when I was fourteen, I spent all the money I'd earned mowing lawns on a set of sailplane lessons with a guy named Gus Street at Strawberry Hill, a little grass strip "airport" just west of Winston-Salem, North Carolina, the town where I grew up. I still remember the feeling of my heart pounding as I pulled the big cherry-red knob that unhooked the rope connecting me to the towplane and banked my sailplane toward the field. It was the first time I had ever felt truly alone and free. Most of my friends got that feeling in cars, but for my money being a thousand feet up in a sailplane beat that thrill a hundred times over.

In college in the 1970s I joined the University of North Carolina sport parachuting (or skydiving) team. It felt like a secret brotherhood—a group of people who knew about something special and magical. My first jump was terrifying, and the second even more so. But by my twelfth jump, when I stepped out the door and had to fall for more than a thousand feet before opening my parachute (my first "ten second delay"), I knew I was home. I made 365 parachute jumps in college and logged more than three and a half hours in free fall, mainly in formations with up to twenty-five fellow jumpers. Although I stopped jumping in 1976, I continued to enjoy vivid dreams about skydiving, which were always pleasant.

The best jumps were often late in the afternoon, when the sun was starting to sink beneath the horizon. It's hard to describe the feeling I would get on those jumps: a feeling of getting close to something that I could never quite name but that I knew I had to have more of. It wasn't solitude exactly, because the way we dived actually wasn't all that solitary. We'd jump five, six, sometimes ten or twelve people at a time, building free-fall formations. The bigger and the more challenging, the better.

One beautiful autumn Saturday in 1975, the rest of the UNC jumpers and I teamed up with some of our friends at a paracenter in eastern North Carolina for some formations. On our penultimate jump of the day, out of a D18 Beechcraft at 10,500 feet, we made a ten-man snowflake. We managed to get ourselves into complete formation before we passed 7,000 feet, and thus were able to enjoy a full eighteen seconds of flying the formation down a clear chasm between two towering cumulus clouds before breaking apart at 3,500 feet and tracking away from each other to open our chutes.

By the time we hit the ground, the sun was down. But by hustling into another plane and taking off again quickly, we managed to get back up into the last of the sun's rays and do a second sunset jump. For this one, two junior members were getting their first shot at flying into formation—that is, joining it from the outside rather than being the base or pin man (which is easier because your job is essentially to fall straight down while everyone else maneuvers toward you). It was exciting for the two junior members, but also for those of us who were more seasoned, because we were building the team, adding to the experience of jumpers who'd later be capable of joining us for even bigger formations.

I was to be the last man out in a six-man star attempt above the runways of the small airport just outside Roanoke Rapids, North Carolina. The guy directly in front of me was named Chuck. Chuck was fairly experienced at "relative work," or RW—that is, building free-fall formations. We were still in sunshine at 7,500 feet, but a mile and a half below us the streetlights were blinking on. Twilight jumps were always sublime and this was clearly going to be a beautiful one.

Even though I'd be exiting the plane a mere second or so behind Chuck, I'd have to move fast to catch up with everyone. I'd rocket straight down headfirst for the first seven seconds or so. This would make me drop almost 100 miles per hour faster than my friends so that I could be right there with them after they had built the initial formation.

Normal procedure for RW jumps was for all jumpers to break apart at 3,500 feet and track away from the formation for maximum separation. Each would then "wave off" with his arms (signaling imminent deployment of his parachute), turn to look above to make sure no others were above him, then pull the rip cord.

"Three, two, one . . . go!"

The first four jumpers exited, then Chuck and I followed close behind. Upside down in a full-head dive and approaching terminal velocity, I smiled as I saw the sun setting for the second time that day. After streaking down to the others, my plan was to slam on the air brakes by throwing out my arms (we had fabric wings from wrists to hips that gave tremendous resistance when fully inflated at high speed) and aiming my jumpsuit's bell-bottomed sleeves and pant legs straight into the oncoming air.

But I never had the chance.

Plummeting toward the formation, I saw that one of the new guys had come in too fast. Maybe falling rapidly between nearby clouds had him a little spooked—it reminded him that he was moving about two hundred feet per second toward that giant planet below, partially shrouded in the gathering darkness. Rather than slowly joining the edge of the formation, he'd barreled in and knocked everybody loose. Now all five other jumpers were tumbling out of control.

They were also much too close together. A skydiver leaves a super-turbulent stream of low-pressure air behind him. If a jumper gets into that trail, he instantly speeds up and can crash into the person below him. That, in turn, can make both jumpers accelerate and slam into anyone who might be below *them*. In short, it's a recipe for disaster.

I angled my body and tracked away from the group to avoid the tumbling mess. I maneuvered until I was falling right over "the spot," a magical point on the ground above which we were to open our parachutes for the leisurely two-minute descent.

I looked over and was relieved to see that the disoriented jumpers were now also tracking away from each other, dispersing the deadly clump.

Chuck was there among them. To my surprise, he was coming straight in my direction. He stopped directly beneath me. With all of the group's tumbling, we were passing through 2,000 feet elevation more quickly than Chuck had anticipated. Maybe he thought he was lucky and didn't have to follow the rules—exactly.

He must not see me. The thought barely had time to go through my head before Chuck's colorful pilot chute blossomed out of his backpack. His pilot chute caught the 120-mph breeze coming around him and shot straight toward me, pulling his main parachute in its sleeve right behind it.

From the instant I saw Chuck's pilot chute emerge, I had a fraction of a second to react. For it would take less than a second to tumble through his deploying main parachute, and—quite likely—right into Chuck himself. At that speed, if I hit his arm or his leg I would take it right off, dealing myself a fatal blow in the process. If I hit him directly, both our bodies would essentially explode.

People say things move more slowly in situations like this, and they're right. My mind watched the action in the microseconds that followed as if it were watching a movie in slow motion.

The instant I saw the pilot chute, my arms flew to my sides and I straightened my body into a head dive, bending ever so slightly at the hips. The verticality gave me increased speed, and the bend allowed my body to add first a little, then a blast of horizontal motion as my body became an efficient wing, sending me zipping past Chuck just in front of his colorful blossoming Para-Commander parachute.

I passed him going at over 150 miles per hour, or 220 feet per second. Given that speed, I doubt he saw the expression on my face. But if he had, he would have seen a look of sheer astonishment. Somehow I had reacted in microseconds to a situation that, had I actually had time to think about it, would have been much too complex for me to deal with.

And yet . . . I *had* dealt with it, and we both landed safely. It was as if, presented with a situation that required more than its usual ability to respond, my brain had become, for a moment, superpowered.

How had I done it? Over the course of my twenty-plus-year career in academic neurosurgery—of studying the brain, observing how it works, and operating on it—I have had plenty of opportunities to ponder this very question. I finally chalked it up to the fact that the brain is truly an extraordinary device: more extraordinary than we can even guess.

I realize now that the real answer to that question is much more profound. But I had to go through a complete metamorphosis of my life and worldview to glimpse that answer. This book is about the events that changed my mind on the matter. They convinced me that, as marvelous a mechanism as the brain is, it was not my brain that saved my life that day at all. What sprang into action the second Chuck's chute started to open was another, much deeper part of me. A part that could move so fast because it was not stuck in time at all, the way the brain and body are.

This was the same part of me, in fact, that had made me so homesick for the skies as a kid. It's not only the smartest part of us, but the deepest part as well, yet for most of my adult life I was unable to believe in it.

But I do believe now, and the pages that follow will tell you why.

I'm a neurosurgeon.

I graduated from the University of North Carolina at Chapel Hill in 1976 with a major in chemistry and earned my M.D. at Duke University Medical School in 1980. During my eleven years of medical school and residency training at Duke as well as Massachusetts General Hospital and Harvard, I focused on neuroendocrinology, the study of the interactions between the nervous system and the endocrine system—the series of glands that release the hormones that direct most of your body's activities. I also spent two of those eleven years investigating how blood vessels in one area of the brain react pathologically when there is bleeding into it from an aneurysm—a syndrome known as cerebral vasospasm.

After completing a fellowship in cerebrovascular neurosurgery in Newcastle-Upon-Tyne in the United Kingdom, I spent fifteen years on the faculty of Harvard Medical School as an associate professor of surgery, with a specialization in neurosurgery. During those years I operated on countless patients, many of them with severe, life-threatening brain conditions.

Most of my research work involved the development of advanced technical procedures like stereotactic radiosurgery, a technique that allows surgeons to precisely guide beams of radiation to specific targets deep in the brain without affecting adjacent areas. I also helped develop magnetic resonance image–guided neurosurgical procedures instrumental in repairing hard-to-treat brain conditions like tumors and vascular disorders.

During those years I also authored or coauthored more than 150 chapters and papers for peer-reviewed medical journals and presented my findings at more than two hundred medical conferences around the world.

In short, I devoted myself to science. Using the tools of modern medicine to help and to heal people, and to learn more about the workings of the human body and brain, was my life's calling. I felt immeasurably lucky to have found it. More important, I had a beautiful wife and two lovely children, and while I was in many ways married to my work, I did not neglect my family, which I considered the other great blessing in my life. On many counts I was a very lucky man, and I knew it.

On November 10, 2008, however, at age fifty-four, my luck seemed to run out. I was struck by a rare illness and thrown into a coma for seven days. During that time, my entire neocortex—the outer surface of the brain, the part that makes us human—was shut down. Inoperative. In essence, absent.

When your brain is absent, you are absent, too. As a neurosurgeon, I'd heard many stories over the years of people who had strange experiences, usually after suffering cardiac arrest: stories of traveling to mysterious, wonderful landscapes; of talking to dead relatives—even of meeting God Himself.

Wonderful stuff, no question. But all of it, in my opinion, was pure fantasy. What caused the otherworldly types of experiences that such people so often report? I didn't claim to know, but I did know that they were brain-based. All of consciousness is. If you don't have a working brain, you can't be conscious.

This is because the brain is the machine that produces consciousness in the first place. When the machine breaks down, consciousness stops. As vastly complicated and mysterious as the actual mechanics of brain processes are, in essence the matter is as simple as that. Pull the plug and the TV goes dead. The show is over, no matter how much you might have been enjoying it.

Or so I would have told you before my own brain crashed.

During my coma my brain wasn't working improperly—it wasn't working *at all*. I now believe that this might have been what was responsible for the depth and intensity of the near-death experience (NDE) that I myself underwent during it. Many of the NDEs reported happen when a person's heart has shut down for a while. In those cases, the neocortex is temporarily inactivated, but generally not too damaged, provided that the flow of oxygenated blood is restored through cardiopulmonary resuscitation or reactivation of cardiac function within four minutes or so. But in my case, the neocortex was out of the picture. I was encountering the reality of a world of consciousness that existed *completely free of the limitations of my physical brain.*

Mine was in some ways a perfect storm of near-death experiences. As a practicing neurosurgeon with decades of research and hands-on work in the operating room behind me, I was in a better-than-average position to judge not only the reality but also the *implications* of what happened to me.

Those implications are tremendous beyond description. My experience showed me that the death of the body and the brain are not the end of consciousness, that human experience continues beyond the grave. More important, it continues under the gaze of a God who loves and cares about each one of us and about where the universe itself and all the beings within it are ultimately going.

The place I went was real. Real in a way that makes the life we're living here and now completely dreamlike by comparison. This doesn't mean I don't value the life I'm living now, however.

In fact, I value it more than I ever did before. I do so because I now see it in its true context.

This life isn't meaningless. But we can't see that fact from here—at least most of the time. What happened to me while I was in that coma is hands-down the most important story I will ever tell. But it's a tricky story to tell because it is so foreign to ordinary understanding. I can't simply shout it from the roof-tops. At the same time, my conclusions are based on a medical analysis of my experience, and on my familiarity with the most advanced concepts in brain science and consciousness studies. Once I realized the truth behind my journey, I knew I *had* to tell it. Doing so properly has become the chief task of my life.

That's not to say I've abandoned my medical work and my life as a neurosurgeon. But now that I have been privileged to understand that our life does not end with the death of the body or the brain, I see it as my duty, my calling, to tell people about what I saw beyond the body and beyond this earth. I am especially eager to tell my story to the people who might have heard stories similar to mine before and wanted to believe them, but had not been able to fully do so.

It is to these people, more than any other, that I direct this book, and the message within it. What I have to tell you is as important as anything anyone will ever tell you, and it's true.

I.

The Pain

Lynchburg, Virginia—November 10, 2008

My eyes popped open. In the darkness of our bedroom, I focused on the red glow of the bedside clock: 4:30 A.M.—an hour before I'd usually wake up for the seventy-minute drive from our house in Lynchburg, Virginia, to the Focused Ultrasound Surgery Foundation in Charlottesville where I worked. My wife, Holley, was still sleeping soundly beside me.

After spending almost twenty years in academic neurosurgery in the greater Boston area, I'd moved with Holley and the rest of our family to the highlands of Virginia two years earlier, in 2006. Holley and I met in October 1977, two years after both of us had left college. Holley was working toward her masters in fine arts, and I was in medical school. She'd been on a couple of dates with my college roommate, Vic. One day, he brought her by to meet me—probably to show her off. As they were leaving, I told Holley to come back anytime, adding that she shouldn't feel obliged to bring Vic.

On our first true date, we drove to a party in Charlotte, North Carolina, two and a half hours each way by car. Holley had laryngitis so I had to do 99 percent of the talking both ways. It was easy. We were married in June 1980 at St Thomas's Episcopal Church in Windsor, North Carolina, and soon after moved into the Royal Oaks apartments in Durham, where I was a resident in surgery at Duke. Our place was far from royal, and I don't recall spotting any oaks there, either. We had very little money but we were both so busy—and so happy to be together—that we didn't care. One of our first vacations was a springtime camping tour of North Carolina's beaches. Spring is no-see-um (the biting midge) bug season in the Carolinas, and our tent didn't offer much protection from them. We had plenty of fun just the same. Swimming in the surf one afternoon at Ocracoke, I devised a way to catch the blue-shell crabs that were scuttling about at my feet. We took a big batch over to the Pony Island Motel, where some friends were staying, and cooked them up on a grill. There was plenty to share with everyone. Despite all our cutting corners, it wasn't long till we found ourselves distressingly low on cash. We were staying with our best friends Bill and Patty Wilson, and, on a whim, decided to accompany them to a night of bingo. Bill had been going every Thursday of every summer for ten years and he had never won. It was Holley's first time playing bingo. Call it beginner's luck, or divine intervention, but she won two hundred dollars—which felt like five thousand dollars to us. The cash extended our trip and made it much more relaxed.

I earned my M.D. in 1980, just as Holley earned her degree and began a career as an artist and teacher. I performed my first solo brain surgery at Duke in 1981. Our firstborn, Eben IV, was born in 1987 at the Princess Mary Maternity Hospital in Newcastle-Upon-Tyne in northern England during my cerebrovascular fellowship, and our younger son, Bond, was born at the Brigham & Women's Hospital in Boston in 1998.

I loved my fifteen years working at Harvard Medical School and Brigham & Women's Hospital. Our family treasured those years in the Greater Boston area. But, in 2005 Holley and I agreed it was time to move back to the South. We wanted to be closer to our families, and I saw it as an opportunity to have a bit more autonomy than I'd had at Harvard. So in the spring of 2006, we started anew in Lynchburg, in the highlands of Virginia. It didn't take long for us to settle back into the more relaxed life we'd both enjoyed growing up in the South.

For a moment I just lay there, vaguely trying to zero in on what had awakened me. The previous day—a Sunday—had been sunny, clear, and just a little crisp—classic late autumn Virginia weather. Holley, Bond (ten years old at the time), and I had gone to a barbecue at the home of a neighbor. In the evening we had spoken by phone to our son Eben IV (then twenty), who was a junior at the University of Delaware. The only hitch in the day had been the mild respiratory virus that Holley, Bond, and I were all still dragging around from the previous week. My back had started aching just before bedtime, so I'd taken a quick bath, which seemed to drive the pain into submission. I wondered if I had awakened so early this morning because the virus was still lurking in my body.

I shifted slightly in bed and a wave of pain shot down my spine—far more intense than the night before. Clearly the flu virus was still hanging on, and then some. The more I awoke, the worse the pain became. Since I wasn't able to fall back to sleep and had an hour to spend before my workday started, I decided on another warm bath. I sat up in bed, swung my feet to the floor, and stood up.

Instantly the pain ratcheted up another notch—a dull, punishing throb penetrating deeply at the base of my spine. Leaving Holley asleep, I padded gingerly down the hall to the main upstairs bathroom.

I ran some water and eased myself into the tub, pretty certain that the warmth would instantly do some good. Wrong. By the time the tub was half full, I knew that I'd made a mistake. Not only was the pain getting worse, but it was also so intense now that I feared I might have to shout for Holley to help me get out of the tub.

Thinking how ridiculous the situation had become, I reached up and grabbed a towel hanging from a rack directly above me. I edged the towel over to the side of the rack so that the rack would be less likely to break loose from the wall and gently pulled myself up.

Another jolt of pain shot down my back, so intense that I gasped. This was definitely *not* the flu. But what else could it be? After struggling out of the slippery tub and into my scarlet terry-cloth bathrobe, I slowly made my way back to our bedroom and flopped down on our bed. My body was already damp again from cold sweat.

Holley stirred and turned over.

"What's going on? What time is it?"

"I don't know," I said. "My back. I am in serious pain."

Holley began rubbing my back. To my surprise it made me feel a little better. Doctors, by and large, don't take kindly to being sick. I'm no exception. For a moment I was convinced the pain—and whatever was causing it—would finally start to recede. But by 6:30 A.M., the time I usually left for work, I was still in agony and virtually paralyzed.

Bond came into our bedroom at 7:30, curious as to why I was still at home.

"What's going on?"

"Your father doesn't feel well, honey," Holley said.

I was still lying on the bed with my head propped up on a

pillow. Bond came over, reached out, and began to massage my temples gently.

His touch sent what felt like a lightning bolt through my head—the worst pain yet. I screamed. Surprised by my reaction, Bond jumped back.

"It's okay," Holley said to Bond, clearly thinking otherwise. "It's nothing you did. Dad has a horrible headache." Then I heard her say, more to herself than to me: "I wonder if I should call an ambulance."

If there's one thing doctors hate even more than being sick, it's being in the emergency room as a patient. I pictured the house filling up with EMTs, the retinue of stock questions, the ride to the hospital, the paperwork . . . I thought at some point I would begin to feel better and regret calling an ambulance in the first place.

"No, it's okay," I said. "It's bad now but it's bound to get better soon. You should probably help Bond get ready for school."

"Eben, I really think—"

"I'll be fine," I interrupted, my face still buried in the pillow. I was still paralyzed by the pain. "Seriously, do *not* call nine-one-one. I'm not that sick. It's just a muscle spasm in my lower back, and a headache."

Reluctantly, Holley took Bond downstairs and fed him some breakfast before sending him up the street to a friend's house to catch a ride to school. As Bond was going out the front door, the thought occurred to me that if this was something serious and I *did* end up in the hospital, I might not see him after school that afternoon. I mustered all my energy and croaked out, "Have a good day at school, Bond."

By the time Holley came back upstairs to check on me, I was

slipping into unconsciousness. Thinking I was napping, she left me to rest and went downstairs to call some of my colleagues, hoping to get their opinions on what might be happening.

Two hours later, feeling she'd let me rest long enough, she came back to check on me. Pushing open our bedroom door, she saw me lying in bed just as before. But looking closer, she saw that my body wasn't relaxed as it had been, but rigid as a board. She turned on the light and saw that I was jerking violently. My lower jaw was jutting forward unnaturally, and my eyes were open and rolling back in my head.

"Eben, say something!" Holley screamed. When I didn't respond, she called nine-one-one. It took the EMTs less than ten minutes to arrive, and they quickly loaded me into an ambulance bound for the Lynchburg General Hospital emergency room.

Had I been conscious, I could have told Holley exactly what I was undergoing there on the bed during those terrifying moments she spent waiting for the ambulance: a full *grand mal* seizure, brought on, no doubt, by some kind of extremely severe shock to my brain.

But of course, I was not able to do that.

For the next seven days, I would be present to Holley and the rest of my family in body alone. I remember nothing of this world during that week and have had to glean from others those parts of this story that occurred during the time I was unconscious. My mind, my spirit—whatever you may choose to call the central, human part of me—was gone.

The Hospital

The Lynchburg General Hospital emergency room is the second-busiest ER in the state of Virginia and is typically in full swing by 9:30 on a weekday morning. That Monday was no exception. Though I spent most of my workdays in Charlottesville, I'd logged plenty of operating time at Lynchburg General, and I knew just about everyone there.

Laura Potter, an ER physician I'd known and worked with closely for almost two years, received the call from the ambulance that a fifty-four-year-old Caucasian male, in *status epilepticus*, was about to arrive in her ER. As she headed down to the ambulance entrance, she ran over the list of possible causes for the incoming patient's condition. It was the same list that I'd have come up with if I had been in her shoes: alcohol withdrawal; drug overdose; hyponatremia (abnormally low sodium level in the blood); stroke; metastatic or primary brain tumor; intraparenchymal hemorrhage (bleeding into the substance of the brain); brain abscess . . . and meningitis.

When the EMTs wheeled me into Major Bay 1 of the ER, I was still convulsing violently, while intermittently groaning and flailing my arms and legs.

It was obvious to Dr. Potter from the way I was raving and writhing around that my brain was under heavy attack. A nurse brought over a crash cart, another drew blood, and a third replaced the first, now empty, intravenous bag that the EMTs had set up at our house before loading me into the ambulance. As they went to work on me, I was squirming like a six-foot fish pulled out of the water. I spouted bursts of garbled, nonsensical sounds and animal-like cries. Just as troubling to Laura as the seizures was that I seemed to show an asymmetry in the motor control of my body. That could mean that not only was my brain under attack but that serious and possibly irreversible brain damage was already under way.

The sight of any patient in such a state takes getting used to, but Laura had seen it all in her many years in the ER. She had never seen one of her fellow physicians delivered into the ER in this condition, however, and looking closer at the contorted, shouting patient on the gurney, she said, almost to herself, "Eben."

Then, more loudly, alerting the other doctors and nurses in the area: "This is Eben Alexander."

Nearby staff who heard her gathered around my stretcher. Holley, who'd been following the ambulance, joined the crowd while Laura reeled off the obligatory questions about the most obvious possible causes for someone in my condition. Was I withdrawing from alcohol? Had I recently ingested any strong hallucinogenic street drugs? Then she went to work trying to bring my seizures to a halt.

In recent months, Eben IV had been putting me through a vigorous conditioning program for a planned father-son climb up Ecuador's 19,300-foot Mount Cotopaxi, which he had climbed the previous February. The program had increased my strength considerably, making it that much more difficult for the orderlies trying to hold me down. Five minutes and 15 milligrams of intravenous diazepam later, I was still delirious and still trying to fight everyone off, but to Dr. Potter's relief I was at least now fighting with both sides of my body. Holley told

Laura about the severe headache I'd been having before I went into seizure, which prompted Dr. Potter to perform a lumbar puncture—a procedure in which a small amount of cerebrospinal fluid is extracted from the base of the spine.

Cerebrospinal fluid is a clear, watery substance that runs along the surface of the spinal cord and coats the brain, cushioning it from impacts. A normal, healthy human body produces about a pint of it a day, and any diminishment in the clarity of the fluid indicates that an infection or hemorrhage has occurred.

Such an infection is called meningitis: the swelling of the meninges, the membranes that line the inside of the spine and skull and that are in direct contact with the cerebrospinal fluid. In four cases out of five a virus causes the disease. Viral meningitis can make a patient quite ill, but it is only fatal in approximately 1 percent of cases. In one case out of five, however, bacteria cause meningitis. Bacteria, being more primitive than viruses, can be a more dangerous foe. Cases of bacterial meningitis are uniformly fatal if untreated. Even when treated rapidly with the appropriate antibiotics, the mortality rate ranges from 15 to 40 percent.

One of the least likely culprits for bacterial meningitis in adults is a very old and very tough bacteria named *Escherichia coli*—better known simply as *E. coli*. No one knows how old *E. coli* is precisely, but estimates hover between three and four billion years. The organism has no nucleus and reproduces by the primitive but extremely efficient process known as asexual binary fission (in other words, by splitting in two). Imagine a cell filled, essentially, with DNA, that can take in nutrients (usually from other cells that it attacks and absorbs) directly through its cellular wall. Then imagine that it can simultaneously copy several strands of DNA and split into two daughter cells every twenty minutes or so. In an hour, you'll have 8 of them. In twelve hours, 69 billion. By hour fifteen, you'll have 35 trillion. This explosive growth only slows when its food begins to run out.

E. coli are also highly promiscuous. They can trade genes with other bacterial species through a process called bacterial conjugation, which allows an E. coli cell to rapidly pick up new traits (such as resistance to a new antibiotic) when needed. This basic recipe for success has kept E. coli on the planet since the earliest days of unicellular life. We all have E. coli bacteria residing within us—mostly in our gastrointestinal tract. Under normal conditions, this poses no threat to us. But when varieties of E. coli that have picked up DNA strands that make them especially aggressive invade the cerebrospinal fluid around the spinal cord and brain, the primitive cells immediately begin devouring the glucose in the fluid, and whatever else is available to consume, including the brain itself.

No one in the ER, at that point, thought I had E. coli meningitis. They had no reason to suspect it. The disease is astronomically rare in adults. Newborns are the most common victims, but cases of babies any older than three months having it are exceedingly uncommon. Fewer than one in 10 million adults contract it spontaneously each year.

In cases of bacterial meningitis, the bacteria attack the outer layer of the brain, or cortex, first. The word *cortex* derives from a Latin word meaning "rind" or "bark." If you picture an orange, its rind is a pretty good model for the way the cortex surrounds the more primitive sections of the brain. The cortex is responsible for memory, language, emotion, visual and auditory awareness, and logic. So when an organism like E. coli attacks the brain, the initial damage is to the areas that perform the functions most crucial to maintaining our human qualities. Many victims of bacterial meningitis die in the first several days of their illness. Of those who arrive in an emergency room with a rapid downward spiral in neurologic function, as I did, only 10 percent are lucky enough to survive. However, their luck is limited, as many of them will spend the rest of their lives in a vegetative state.

Though she didn't suspect *E. coli* meningitis, Dr. Potter thought I might have *some* kind of brain infection, which is why she decided on the lumbar puncture. Just as she was telling one of the nurses to bring her a lumbar puncture tray and prepare me for the procedure, my body surged up as if my gurney had been electrified. With a fresh blast of energy, I let out a long, agonized groan, arched my back, and flailed my arms at the air. My face was red, and the veins in my neck bulged out crazily. Laura shouted for more help, and soon two, then four, and finally six attendants were struggling to hold me down for the procedure. They forced my body into a fetal position while Laura administered more sedatives. Finally, they were able to make me still enough for the needle to penetrate the base of my spine.

When bacteria attack, the body goes immediately into defense mode, sending shock troops of white blood cells from their barracks in the spleen and bone marrow to fight off the invaders. They're the first casualties in the massive cellular war that happens whenever a foreign biological agent invades the body, and Dr. Potter knew that any lack of clarity in my cerebrospinal fluid would be caused by my white blood cells.

Dr. Potter bent over and focused on the manometer, the transparent vertical tube into which the cerebrospinal fluid would emerge. Laura's first surprise was that the fluid didn't drip but gushed out—due to dangerously high pressure.

Her second surprise was the fluid's appearance. The slightest opacity would tell her I was in deep trouble. What shot out into the manometer was viscous and white, with a subtle tinge of green.

My spinal fluid was full of pus.

3

Out of Nowhere

Dr. Potter paged Dr. Robert Brennan, one of her associates at Lynchburg General and a specialist in infectious disease. While they waited for more test results to come from the adjacent labs, they considered all of the diagnostic possibilities and therapeutic options.

Minute by minute, as the test results came back, I continued to groan and squirm beneath the straps on my gurney. An ever more baffling picture was emerging. The Gram's stain (a chemical test, named after a Danish physician who invented the method, that allows doctors to classify an invading bacteria as either gram-negative or gram-positive) came back indicating gram-negative rods—which was highly unusual.

Meanwhile a computerized tomography (CT) scan of my head showed that the meningeal lining of my brain was dangerously swollen and inflamed. A breathing tube was put into my trachea, allowing a ventilator to take over the job of breathing for me—twelve breaths a minute, exactly—and a battery of monitors was set up around my bed to record every movement within my body and my now all-but-destroyed brain.

Of the very few adults who contract spontaneous *E. coli* bacterial meningitis (that is, without brain surgery or penetrating head trauma) each year, most do so because of some tangible cause, such as a deficiency in their immune system (often caused by HIV or AIDS). But I had no such factor that would have made me susceptible to the disease. Other bacteria might cause meningitis by invading from the adjacent nasal sinuses or middle ear, but not *E. coli*. The cerebrospinal space is too well sealed off from the rest of the body for that to happen. Unless the spine or skull is punctured (by a contaminated deep brain stimulator or a shunt installed by a neurosurgeon, for example), bacteria like *E. coli* that usually reside in the gut simply have no access to that area. I had installed hundreds of shunts and stimulators in the brains of patients myself, and had I been able to discuss the matter, I would have agreed with my stumped doctors that, to put it simply, I had a disease that was virtually impossible for me to have.

Still unable to completely accept the evidence being presented from the test results, the two doctors placed calls to experts in infectious disease at major academic medical centers. Everyone agreed that the results pointed to only one possible diagnosis.

But contracting a case of severe *E. coli* bacterial meningitis out of thin air was not the only strange medical feat I performed that first day in the hospital. In the final moments before leaving the emergency room, and after two straight hours of guttural animal wails and groaning, I became quiet. Then, out of nowhere, I shouted three words. They were crystal clear, and heard by all the doctors and nurses present, as well as by Holley, who stood a few paces away, just on the other side of the curtain.

"God, help me!"

Everyone rushed over to the stretcher. By the time they got to me, I was completely unresponsive.

I have no memory of my time in the ER, including those three words I shouted out. But they were the last I would speak for the next seven days.

4

Eben IV

Once in Major Bay 1, I continued to decline. The cerebrospinal fluid (CSF) glucose level of a normal healthy person is around 80 milligrams per deciliter. An extremely sick person in imminent danger of dying from bacterial meningitis can have a level as low as 20 mg/dl.

I had a CSF glucose level of 1. My Glasgow Coma Scale was eight out of fifteen, indicative of a severe brain illness, and declined further over the next few days. My APACHE II score (Acute Physiology and Chronic Health Evaluation) in the ER was 18 out of a possible 71, indicating that the chances of my dying during that hospitalization were about 30 percent. More specifically, given my diagnosis of acute gram-negative bacterial meningitis and rapid neurological decline at the outset, I'd had, at best, only about a 10 percent chance of surviving my illness when I was admitted to the ER. If the antibiotics didn't kick in, the risk of mortality would rise steadily over the next few days—till it hit a nonnegotiable 100 percent.

The doctors loaded my body with three powerful intravenous antibiotics before sending me up to my new home: a large private room, number 10, in the Medical Intensive Care Unit, one floor above the ER.

I'd been in these ICUs many times as a surgeon. They are where the absolute sickest patients, people just inches from death, are placed, so that several medical personnel can work on them simultaneously. A team like that, fighting in complete coordination to keep a patient alive when all the odds are against them, is an awesome sight. I had felt both enormous pride and brutal disappointment in those rooms, depending on whether the patient we were struggling to save either made it or slipped from our fingers.

Dr. Brennan and the rest of the doctors stayed as upbeat with Holley as they could, given the circumstances. This didn't allow for their being at all upbeat. The truth was that I was at significant risk of dying, very soon. Even if I didn't die, the bacteria attacking my brain had probably already devoured enough of my cortex to compromise any higher-brain activity. The longer I stayed in coma, the more likely it became that I would spend the rest of my life in a chronic vegetative state.

Fortunately, not only the staff of Lynchburg General but other people, too, were already gathering to help. Michael Sullivan, our neighbor and the rector in our Episcopal church, arrived at the ER about an hour after Holley. Just as Holley had run out the door to follow the ambulance, her cell phone had buzzed. It was her longtime friend Sylvia White. Sylvia always had an uncanny way of reaching out precisely when important things were happening. Holley was convinced she was psychic. (I had opted for the safer and more sensible explanation that she was just a very good guesser.) Holley briefed Sylvia on what was happening, and between them they made calls to my immediate family: my younger sister, Betsy, who lived nearby, my sister Phyllis, at forty-eight the youngest of us, who was living in Boston, and Jean, the oldest.

That Monday morning Jean was driving south through Virginia from her home in Delaware. Fortuitously, she was on her way to help our mother, who lived in Winston-Salem. Jean's cell phone rang. It was her husband, David.

"Have you gone through Richmond yet?" he asked.

"No," Jean said. "I'm just north of it on I-95."

"Get onto route 60 West, then route 24 down to Lynchburg. Holley just called. Eben's in the emergency room there. He had a seizure this morning and isn't responding."

"Oh, my God! Do they have any idea why?"

"They're not sure, but it might be meningitis."

Jean made the turn just in time and followed the undulating two-lane blacktop of 60 West through low, scudding clouds, toward Route 24 and Lynchburg.

It was Phyllis who, at three o'clock that first afternoon of the emergency, called Eben IV at his apartment at the University of Delaware. Eben was outside on his porch doing some science homework (my own dad had been a neurosurgeon, and Eben was interested in that career now as well) when his phone rang. Phyllis gave him a quick rundown of the situation and told him not to worry—that the doctors had everything under control.

"Do they have any idea what it might be?" Eben asked.

"Well, they did mention gram-negative bacteria and meningitis."

"I have two exams in the next few days, so I'm going to leave some quick messages with my teachers," said Eben.

Eben later told me that, initially, he was hesitant to believe that I was in as grave danger as Phyllis had indicated, since she and Holley always "blew things out of proportion"—*and* I never got sick. But when Michael Sullivan called him on the phone an hour later, he realized that he needed to make the drive down— *immediately.*

As Eben drove toward Virginia, an icy pelting rain started up. Phyllis had left Boston at six o'clock, and as Eben headed toward the I-495 bridge over the Potomac River into Virginia, she was passing through the clouds overhead. She landed at Richmond, rented a car, and got onto Route 60 herself.

When he was just a few miles outside Lynchburg, Eben called Holley.

"How's Bond?" he asked.

"Asleep," Holley said.

"I'm going to go straight to the hospital then," Eben said.

"You sure you don't want to come home first?"

"No," Eben said. "I just want to see Dad."

Eben pulled up at the Medical Intensive Care Unit at 11:15 P.M. The walkway into the hospital was starting to ice over, and when he came into the bright lights of the reception area he saw only a night reception nurse. She led him to my ICU bed.

By that point, everyone who had been there earlier had finally gone home. The only sounds in the large, dimly lit room were the quiet beeps and hisses of the machines keeping my body going.

Eben froze in the doorway when he saw me. In his twenty years, he'd never seen me with more than a cold. Now, in spite of all the machines doing their best to make it seem otherwise, he was looking at what he knew was, essentially, a corpse. My physical body was there in front of him, but the dad he knew was gone.

Or perhaps a better word to use is: elsewhere.

5.

Underworld

Darkness, but a visible darkness—like being submerged in mud yet also being able to see through it. Or maybe dirty Jell-O describes it better. Transparent, but in a bleary, blurry, claustrophobic, suffocating kind of way.

Consciousness, but consciousness without memory or identity—like a dream where you know what's going on around you, but have no real idea of who, or what, *you* are.

Sound, too: a deep, rhythmic pounding, distant yet strong, so that each pulse of it goes right through you. Like a heartbeat? A little, but darker, more mechanical—like the sound of metal against metal, as if a giant, subterranean blacksmith is pounding an anvil somewhere off in the distance: pounding it so hard that the sound vibrates through the earth, or the mud, or wherever it is that you are.

I didn't have a body—not one that I was aware of anyway. I was simply . . . *there*, in this place of pulsing, pounding darkness. At the time, I might have called it "primordial." But at the time it was going on, I didn't know this word. In fact, I didn't know any words at all. The words used here registered much later, when, back in the world, I was writing down my recollections. Language, emotion, logic: these were all gone, as if I had regressed back to some state of being from the very beginnings of life, as far back, perhaps, as the primitive bacteria that, unbeknownst to me, had taken over my brain and shut it down.

How long did I reside in this world? I have no idea. When

you go to a place where there's no sense of time as we experience it in the ordinary world, accurately describing the way it feels is next to impossible. When it was happening, when I was there, I felt like I (whatever "I" was) had always been there and would always continue to be.

Nor, initially at least, did I mind this. Why would I, after all, since this state of being was the only one I'd ever known? Having no memory of anything better, I was not particularly bothered by where I was. I do recall conceptualizing that I might or might not survive, but my indifference as to whether I did or not only gave me a greater feeling of invulnerability. I was clueless as to the rules that governed this world I was in, but I was in no hurry to learn them. After all, why bother?

I can't say exactly when it happened, but at a certain point I became aware of some objects around me. They were a little like roots, and a little like blood vessels in a vast, muddy womb. Glowing a dark, dirty red, they reached down from some place far above to some other place equally far below. In retrospect, looking at them was like being a mole or earthworm, buried deep in the ground yet somehow able to see the tangled matrixes of roots and trees surrounding it.

That's why, thinking back to this place later, I came to call it the Realm of the Earthworm's-Eye View. For a long time, I suspected it might have been some kind of memory of what my brain felt like during the period when the bacteria were originally overrunning it.

But the more I thought about this explanation (and again, this was all much, much later), the less sense it made. Because—hard as this is to picture if you haven't been to this place yourself—my consciousness wasn't foggy or distorted when I was there. It was just . . . *limited*. I wasn't human while I was in this place. I wasn't even animal. I was something before, and below, all that. I was simply a lone point of awareness in a time-less red-brown sea.

The longer I stayed in this place, the less comfortable I be-came. At first I was so deeply immersed in it that there was no difference between "me" and the half-creepy, half-familiar element that surrounded me. But gradually this sense of deep, timeless, and boundaryless immersion gave way to something else: a feeling like I wasn't really part of this subterranean world at all, but trapped in it.

Grotesque animal faces bubbled out of the muck, groaned or screeched, and then were gone again. I heard an occasional dull roar. Sometimes these roars changed to dim, rhythmic chants, chants that were both terrifying and weirdly familiar—as if at some point I'd known and uttered them all myself.

As I had no memory of prior existence, my time in this realm stretched way, way out. Months? Years? Eternity? Regardless of the answer, I eventually got to a point where the creepy-crawly feeling totally outweighed the homey, familiar feeling. The more I began to feel like a *me*—like something separate from the cold and wet and dark around me—the more the faces that bubbled up out of that darkness became ugly and threatening. The rhyth-mic pounding off in the distance sharpened and intensified as well—became the work-beat for some army of troll-like under-ground laborers, performing some endless, brutally monotonous task. The movement around me became less visual and more tactile, as if reptilian, wormlike creatures were crowding past, occasionally rubbing up against me with their smooth or spiky skins.

Then I became aware of a smell: a little like feces, a little like blood, and a little like vomit. A *biological* smell, in other words,

but of biological death, not of biological life. As my awareness sharpened more and more, I edged ever closer to panic.
Whoever or whatever I was, I did not belong here. I needed to
get out.

But where would I go?

Even as I asked that question, something new emerged from
the darkness above: something that wasn't cold, or dead, or dark,
but the exact opposite of all those things. If I tried for the rest
of my life, I would never be able to do justice to this entity that
now approached me ... to come anywhere close to describing
how beautiful it was.

But I'm going to try.

6.

An Anchor to Life

Phyllis pulled into the hospital parking lot just under two hours after Eben IV had, at around 1 A.M. When she got to my ICU room she found Eben IV sitting next to my bed, clutching a hospital pillow in front of him to help him keep awake.

"Mom's home with Bond," Eben said, in a tone that was tired, tense, and happy to see her, all at once.

Phyllis told Eben he needed to go home, that if he stayed up all night after driving from Delaware he'd be worthless to anyone tomorrow, his dad included. She called Holley and Jean at our house and told them Eben IV would be back soon but that she was staying in my room for the night.

"Go home to your mom and your aunt and your brother," she said to Eben IV when she'd hung up. "They need you. Your dad and I will be right here when you get back tomorrow."

Eben IV looked over at my body: at the clear plastic breathing tube running through my right nostril down to my trachea; at my thin, already chapping lips; at my closed eyes and sagging facial muscles.

Phyllis read his thoughts.

"Go home, Eben. Try not to worry. Your dad's still with us. And I'm not going to let him go."

She walked to my bedside, picked up my hand, and started to massage it. With only the machines and the night nurse who came in to check my stats every hour for company, Phyllis sat through the rest of the night, holding my hand, keeping a connection going that she knew full well was vital if I was going to get through this.

It's a cliché to talk about what a big emphasis people in the South put on family, but like a lot of clichés, it's also true. When I went to Harvard in 1988, one of the first things I noticed about northerners was the way they were a little shyer about expressing a fact that many in the South take for granted: Your family is *who you are.*

Throughout my own life, my relationship with my family—with my parents and sisters, and later with Holley, Eben IV, and Bond—had always been a vital source of strength and stability, but even more so in recent years. Family was where I turned for unquestioning support in a world that—North or South—can all too often be short of this commodity.

I went to our Episcopal church with Holley and the kids on occasion. But the fact was that for years I'd only been a step above a "C & E'er" (one who only darkens the door of a church at Christmas and Easter). I encouraged our boys to say their prayers at night, but I was no spiritual leader in our home. I'd never escaped my feelings of doubt at how any of it could really *be.* As much as I'd grown up wanting to believe in God and Heaven and an afterlife, my decades in the rigorous scientific world of academic neurosurgery had profoundly called into question how such things could exist. Modern neuroscience dictates that the brain gives rise to consciousness—to the mind, to the soul, to the spirit, to whatever you choose to call that invisible, intangible part of us that truly makes us who we are—and I had little doubt that it was correct.

Like most health-care workers who deal directly with dying patients and their families, I had heard about—and even seen—

some pretty inexplicable events over the years. I filed those occurrences under "unknown" and let them be, figuring a commonsense answer of one kind or another lay at the heart of them all.

Not that I was opposed to supernatural beliefs. As a doctor who saw incredible physical and emotional suffering on a regular basis, the last thing I would have wanted to do was to deny anyone the comfort and hope that faith provided. In fact, I would have loved to have enjoyed some of it myself.

The older I got, however, the less likely that seemed. Like an ocean wearing away a beach, over the years my scientific worldview gently but steadily undermined my ability to believe in something larger. Science seemed to be providing a steady onslaught of evidence that pushed our significance in the universe ever closer to zero. Belief would have been nice. But science is not concerned with what would be nice. It's concerned with what *is*.

I'm a kinetic learner, which is just to say that I learn by doing. If I can't feel something or touch it myself, it's hard for me to take interest in it. That desire to reach out and touch whatever I'm trying to understand was, along with the desire to be like my father, what drew me to neurosurgery. As abstract and mysterious as the human brain is, it's also incredibly concrete. As a medical student at Duke, I relished looking into a microscope and actually seeing the delicately elongated neuronal cells that spark the synaptic connections that give rise to consciousness. I loved the combination of abstract knowledge and total physicality that brain surgery presented. To access the brain, one must pull away the layers of skin and tissue covering the skull and apply a high-speed pneumatic device called a Midas Rex drill. It's a very sophisticated piece of equipment, costing thousands of dollars. Yet when you get down to it, it's also just . . . a drill.

Likewise, surgically repairing the brain, while an extraordinarily complex undertaking, is actually no different than fixing any other highly delicate, electrically charged machine. That, I knew full well, is what the brain really is: a machine that produces the phenomenon of consciousness. Sure, scientists hadn't discovered exactly how the neurons of the brain managed to do this, but it was only a matter of time before they would. This was proven every day in the operating room. A patient comes in with headaches and diminished consciousness. You obtain an MRI (magnetic resonance image) of her brain and discover a tumor. You place the patient under general anesthesia, remove the tumor, and a few hours later she's waking up to the world again. No more headaches. No more trouble with consciousness. Seemingly pretty simple.

I adored that simplicity—the absolute honesty and *cleanness* of science. I respected that it left no room for fantasy or for sloppy thinking. If a fact could be established as tangible and trustworthy, it was accepted. If not, then it was rejected.

This approach left very little room for the soul and the spirit, for the continuing existence of a personality after the brain that supported it stopped functioning. It left even less room for those words I'd heard in church again and again: "life everlasting."

Which is why I counted on my family—on Holley and our boys and my three sisters and, of course, my mom and dad—so much. In a very real sense, I'd never have been able to practice my profession—to perform, day in and day out, the actions I performed, and to see the things I saw—without the bedrock support of love and understanding they provided.

And that was why Phyllis (after consulting our sister Betsy on the phone) decided that night to make a promise to me on behalf of our whole family. As she sat there with my limp, nearly lifeless hand in hers, she told me that no matter what happened from then on, someone would always be right there, holding my hand.

"We are not letting you go, Eben," she said. "You need an anchor to keep you here, in this world, where we need you. And we'll provide it."

Little did she know just how important that anchor was going to prove in the days to come.

7

The Spinning Melody and the Gateway

S omething had appeared in the darkness.
Turning slowly, it radiated fine filaments of white-gold light, and as it did so the darkness around me began to splinter and break apart.

Then I heard a new sound: a *living* sound, like the richest, most complex, most beautiful piece of music you've ever heard. Growing in volume as a pure white light descended, it obliterated the monotonous mechanical pounding that, seemingly for eons, had been my only company up until then.

The light got closer and closer, spinning around and around and generating those filaments of pure white light that I now saw were tinged, here and there, with hints of gold.

Then, at the very center of the light, something else appeared. I focused my awareness, hard, trying to figure out what it was.

An opening. I was no longer looking *at* the slowly spinning light at all, but *through* it.

The moment I understood this, I began to move up. Fast. There was a whooshing sound, and in a flash I went through the opening and found myself in a completely new world. The strangest, most beautiful world I'd ever seen.

Brilliant, vibrant, ecstatic, stunning . . . I could heap on one adjective after another to describe what this world looked and felt like, but they'd all fall short. I felt like I was being born. Not reborn, or born again. Just . . . born.

Below me there was countryside. It was green, lush, and

earthlike. It *was* earth . . . but at the same time it wasn't. It was like when your parents take you back to a place where you spent some years as a very young child. You don't know the place. Or at least you think you don't. But as you look around, something pulls at you, and you realize that a part of yourself—a part way, deep down—does remember the place after all, and is rejoicing at being back there again.

I was flying, passing over trees and fields, streams and water-falls, and here and there, people. There were children, too, laughing and playing. The people sang and danced around in circles, and sometimes I'd see a dog, running and jumping among them, as full of joy as the people were. They wore simple yet beautiful clothes, and it seemed to me that the colors of these clothes had the same kind of living warmth as the trees and the flowers that bloomed and blossomed in the countryside around them.

A beautiful, incredible dream world . . .

Except it wasn't a dream. Though I didn't know where I was or even *what* I was, I was absolutely sure of one thing: this place I'd suddenly found myself in was completely real.

The word *real* expresses something abstract, and it's frus-tratingly ineffective at conveying what I'm trying to describe. Imagine being a kid and going to a movie on a summer day. Maybe the movie was good, and you were entertained as you sat through it. But then the show ended, and you filed out of the theater and back into the deep, vibrant, welcoming warmth of the summer afternoon. And as the air and the sunlight hit you, you wondered why on earth you'd wasted this gorgeous day sit-ting in a dark theater.

Multiply that feeling a thousand times, and you still won't be anywhere close to what it felt like where I was.

I don't know how long, exactly, I flew along. (Time in this

place was different from the simple linear time we experience on earth and is as hopelessly difficult to describe as every other aspect of it.) But at some point, I realized that I wasn't alone up there.

Someone was next to me: a beautiful girl with high cheekbones and deep blue eyes. She was wearing the same kind of peasant-like clothes that the people in the village down below wore. Golden-brown tresses framed her lovely face. We were riding along together on an intricately patterned surface, alive with indescribable and vivid colors—the wing of a butterfly. In fact, millions of butterflies were all around us—vast fluttering waves of them, dipping down into the greenery and coming back up around us again. It wasn't any single, discrete butterfly that appeared, but all of them together, as if they were a river of life and color, moving through the air. We flew in lazy looped formations past blossoming flowers and buds on trees that opened as we flew near.

The girl's outfit was simple, but its colors—powder blue, indigo, and pastel orange-peach—had the same overwhelming, super-vivid aliveness that everything else in the surroundings had. She looked at me with a look that, if you saw it for a few moments, would make your whole life up to that point worth living, no matter what had happened in it so far. It was not a romantic look. It was not a look of friendship. It was a look that was somehow beyond all these . . . beyond all the different types of love we have down here on earth. It was something higher, holding all those other kinds of love within itself while at the same time being more genuine and pure than all of them.

Without using any words, she spoke to me. The message went through me like a wind, and I instantly understood that it was true. I knew so in the same way that I knew that the world around us was real—was not some fantasy, passing and insubstantial.

The message had three parts, and if I had to translate them into earthly language, I'd say they ran something like this:

"You are loved and cherished, dearly, forever."

"You have nothing to fear."

"There is nothing you can do wrong."

The message flooded me with a vast and crazy sensation of relief. It was like being handed the rules to a game I'd been playing all my life without ever fully understanding it.

"We will show you many things here," the girl said—again, without actually using these words but by driving their conceptual essence directly into me. "But eventually, you will go back."

To this, I had only one question.

Back where?

Remember who's talking to you right now. I'm not a soft-headed sentimentalist. I know what death looks like. I know what it feels like to have a living person, whom you spoke to and joked with in better days, become a lifeless object on an operating table after you've struggled for hours to keep the machine of their body working. I know what suffering looks like, and the answerless grief on the faces of loved ones who have lost someone they never dreamed they could lose. I know my biology, and while I'm not a physicist, I'm no slouch at that, either. I know the difference between fantasy and reality, and I know that the experience I'm struggling to give you the vaguest, most completely unsatisfactory picture of, was the single most real experience of my life.

In fact, the only competition for it in the reality department was what came next.

8.

Israel

By eight the next morning, Holley was back in my room. She spelled Phyllis, taking her place in the chair by the head of my bed and squeezing my still unresponsive hand in hers. Around 11 A.M., Michael Sullivan arrived, and everyone formed a circle around me, with Betsy holding my hand so that I was included, too. Michael led a prayer. They were just finishing when one of the doctors specializing in infectious diseases came in with a fresh report from downstairs. Despite their adjusting my antibiotics overnight, my white blood cell count was still rising. The bacteria were continuing, unimpeded, with the task of eating my brain.

Fast running out of options, the doctors once more went over the details of my activities in the past few days with Holley. Then they stretched their questions to cover the past few weeks. Was there anything—*anything*—in the details of what I'd been doing that could help them make sense of my condition?

"Well," said Holley, "he did take a work trip to Israel a few months ago."

Dr. Brennan looked up from his notepad.

E. coli bacterial cells can swap DNA not only with other *E. coli*, but with other gram-negative bacterial organisms as well. This has enormous implications in our time of global travel, antibiotic bombardment, and fast-mutating new strains of bacterial illnesses. If some *E. coli* bacteria find themselves in a harsh biological environment with some other primitive organisms that are better suited than they are, the *E. coli* can potentially pick up some DNA from those better-suited bacteria and incorporate it.

In 1996, doctors discovered a new bacterial strain harboring DNA for a gene coding for *Klebsiella pneumoniae* carbapenemase, or KPC, an enzyme that conferred antibiotic resistance on its host bacterium. It was found in the stomach of a patient who died in a North Carolina hospital. The strain immediately got the attention of doctors all over the world when it was discovered that KPC could potentially render a bacteria that absorbed it resistant not just to some current antibiotics, but to *all* of them.

If a toxic, antibiotic-proof strain of bacteria (one whose nontoxic cousin is ubiquitous in our bodies) got loose in the general population, it would have a field day with the human race. There are no new antibiotics in the ten-year pharmaceutical development pipeline that could come to the rescue.

Just a few months earlier, Dr. Brennan knew, a patient had checked into a hospital with a powerful bacterial infection and was given a range of powerful antibiotics in an effort to control his *Klebsiella pneumoniae* infection. But the man's condition continued to worsen. Tests revealed that he was still suffering from *Klebsiella pneumoniae* and that the antibiotics hadn't done their work. Further tests revealed that the bacteria living in the man's large intestine had acquired the KPC gene by direct plasmid transfer from his resistant *Klebsiella pneumoniae* infection. In other words, his body had provided the laboratory for the creation of a species of bacteria that, if it got into the general population, might rival the Black Death, a plague that killed off half of Europe in the fourteenth century.

The hospital where all this occurred was the Sourasky Medical Center in Tel Aviv, Israel, and it had occurred just a few months previously. As a matter of fact it happened at about the time that I'd been there, as part of my work coordinating a global research initiative in focused ultrasound brain surgery. I'd arrived in Jerusalem at 3:15 A.M. and after finding my hotel had decided on a whim to walk to the old city. I ended up taking a lone predawn tour of the Via Dolorosa and visiting the alleged site of the Last Supper. The trip had been strangely moving, and once back in the States I'd often brought it up with Holley. But at the time I'd known nothing of the patient at the Sourasky Medical Center, or the bacteria he contracted that picked up the KPC gene. Bacteria that, it developed, was itself a strain of *E. coli*.

Could I have somehow picked up an antibiotic-proof KPC-harboring bacteria while I was over in Israel? It was unlikely. But it was a possible explanation for the apparent resistance of my infection, and my doctors went to work to determine if that was indeed the bacteria that was attacking my brain. My case was about to become, for the first of many reasons, a part of medical history.

9.

The Core

Meanwhile, I was in a place of clouds.

Big, puffy, pink-white ones that showed up sharply against the deep blue-black sky.

Higher than the clouds—immeasurably higher—flocks of transparent orbs, shimmering beings arced across the sky, leaving long, streamer-like lines behind them.

Birds? Angels? These words registered when I was writing down my recollections. But neither of these words do justice to the beings themselves, which were quite simply different from anything I have known on this planet. They were more advanced. *Higher*.

A sound, huge and booming like a glorious chant, came down from above, and I wondered if the winged beings were producing it. Again thinking about it later, it occurred to me that the joy of these creatures, as they soared along, was such that they *had* to make this noise—that if the joy didn't come out of them this way then they would simply not otherwise be able to contain it. The sound was palpable and almost material, like a rain that you can feel on your skin but that doesn't get you wet.

Seeing and hearing were not separate in this place where I now was. I could *hear* the visual beauty of the silvery bodies of those scintillating beings above, and I could see the surging, joyful perfection of what they sang. It seemed that you could not look at or listen to anything in this world without becoming a part of it—without joining with it in some mysterious way.

Again, from my present perspective, I would suggest that you couldn't look *at* anything in that world at all, for the word *at* itself implies a separation that did not exist there. Everything was distinct, yet everything was also a part of everything else, like the rich and intermingled designs on a Persian carpet ... or a butterfly's wing.

A warm wind blew through, like the kind that spring up on the most perfect summer days, tossing the leaves of the trees and flowing past like heavenly water. A divine breeze. It changed everything, shifting the world around me into an even higher octave, a higher vibration.

Although I still had little language function, at least as we think of it on earth, I began wordlessly putting questions to this wind—and to the divine being that I sensed at work behind or within it.

Where is this place?

Who am I?

Why am I here?

Each time I silently posed one of these questions, the answer came instantly in an explosion of light, color, love, and beauty that blew through me like a crashing wave. What was important about these bursts was that they didn't simply silence my questions by overwhelming them. They *answered* them, but in a way that bypassed language. Thoughts entered me directly. But it wasn't thought like we experience on earth. It wasn't vague, immaterial, or abstract. These thoughts were solid and immediate—hotter than fire and wetter than water—and as I received them I was able to instantly and effortlessly understand concepts that would have taken me years to fully grasp in my earthly life.

I continued moving forward and found myself entering an

immense void, completely dark, infinite in size, yet also infinitely comforting. Pitch black as it was, it was also brimming over with light: a light that seemed to come from a brilliant orb that I now sensed near me. An orb that was living and almost solid, as the songs of the angel beings had been.

My situation was, strangely enough, something akin to that of a fetus in a womb. The fetus floats in the womb with the silent partner of the placenta, which nourishes it and mediates its relationship to the everywhere present yet at the same time invisible mother. In this case, the "mother" was God, the Creator, the Source who is responsible for making the universe and all in it. This Being was so close that there seemed to be no distance at all between God and myself. Yet at the same time, I could sense the infinite vastness of the Creator, could see how completely minuscule I was by comparison. I will occasionally use *Om* as the pronoun for God because I originally used that name in my writings after my coma. "Om" was the sound I remembered hearing associated with that omniscient, omnipotent, and unconditionally loving God, but any descriptive word falls short.

The pure vastness separating Om and me was, I realized, why I had the Orb as my companion. In some manner I couldn't completely comprehend but was sure of nonetheless, the Orb was a kind of "interpreter" between me and this extraordinary presence surrounding me.

It was as if I were being born into a larger world, and the universe itself was like a giant cosmic womb, and the Orb (who remained in some way connected to the Girl on the Butterfly Wing, who in fact *was* she) was guiding me through this process.

Later, when I was back here in the world, I found a quotation by the seventeenth-century Christian poet Henry Vaughan that came close to describing this place—this vast, inky-black core that was the home of the Divine itself.

"There is, some say, in God a deep but dazzling darkness . . ."

That was it, exactly: an inky darkness that was also full to brimming with light.

The questions, and the answers, continued. Though they still didn't come in the form of language as we know it, the "voice" of this Being was warm and—odd as I know this may sound—personal. It understood humans, and it possessed the qualities we possess, only in infinitely greater measure. It knew me deeply and overflowed with qualities that all my life I've always associated with human beings, and human beings alone: warmth, compassion, pathos . . . even irony and humor.

Through the Orb, Om told me that there is not one universe but many—in fact, more than I could conceive—but that love lay at the center of them all. Evil was present in all the other universes as well, but only in the tiniest trace amounts. Evil was necessary because without it free will was impossible, and without free will there could be no growth—no forward movement, no chance for us to become what God longed for us to be. Horrible and all-powerful as evil sometimes seemed to be in a world like ours, in the larger picture love was overwhelmingly dominant, and it would ultimately be triumphant.

I saw the abundance of life throughout the countless universes, including some whose intelligence was advanced far beyond that of humanity. I saw that there are countless higher dimensions, but that the only way to know these dimensions is to enter and experience them directly. They cannot be known, or understood, from lower dimensional space. Cause and effect exist in these higher realms, but outside of our earthly conception of them. The world of time and space in which we move in this terrestrial realm is tightly and intricately meshed within these higher worlds. In other words, these worlds aren't totally apart from us, because all worlds are part of the same overarching divine Reality. From those higher worlds one could access any time or place in our world.

It will take me the rest of my life, and then some, to unpack what I learned up there. The knowledge given me was not "taught" in the way that a history lesson or math theorem would be. Insights happened directly, rather than needing to be coaxed and absorbed. Knowledge was stored without memorization, instantly and for good. It didn't fade, like ordinary information does, and to this day I still possess all of it, much more clearly than I possess the information that I gained over all of my years in school.

That's not to say that I can get to this knowledge just like that. Because now that I'm back here in the earthly realm, I have to process it through my limited physical body and brain. But it's there. I feel it, laid into my very being. For a person like me who had spent his whole life working hard to accumulate knowledge and understanding the old-fashioned way, the discovery of this more advanced level of learning was, alone, enough to give me food for thought for ages to come . . .

Unfortunately, for my family and my doctors back on earth, the situation was very different.

10

What Counts

Holley didn't fail to notice how interested the doctors became when she mentioned my trip to Israel. But of course she didn't understand *why* it was so important. In retrospect, it was a blessing that she didn't. Coping with my possible death was burden enough, without the added possibility that I was the index case for the twenty-first-century equivalent of the Black Plague.

Meanwhile, more calls went out to friends and family.

Including to my biological family.

As a young boy, I'd worshipped my father, who was chief of staff for twenty years at Wake Forest Baptist Medical Center in Winston-Salem. I chose academic neurosurgery as a career in order to follow in his footsteps as closely as I could—despite knowing I'd never completely fill his shoes.

My father was a deeply spiritual man. He served as a surgeon in the Army Air Force in the jungles of New Guinea and the Philippines during World War II. He witnessed brutality and suffering and suffered himself. He told me about nights spent operating on battle casualties in tents that barely held up under the blankets of monsoon rain hitting them, the heat and humidity so oppressive that the surgeons stripped down to their underwear just to be able to endure it.

Dad had married the love of his life (and his commanding officer's daughter), Betty, in October 1942, while training for his stint in the Pacific Theater. At war's end he was part of the initial group of Allied forces occupying Japan after the United States dropped atomic bombs on Hiroshima and Nagasaki. As the only U.S. military neurosurgeon in Tokyo, he was officially indispensable. He was qualified to perform ear, nose, and throat surgery to boot.

All of these qualifications ensured that he would not be going anywhere for quite some time. His new commanding officer would not allow him to go back to the States until the situation was "more stable." Several months after the Japanese formally surrendered aboard the battleship *Missouri* in Tokyo Bay, Dad, at last, received general orders releasing him to go home. However, he knew that the on-site CO would have these orders rescinded if he saw them. So Dad waited until the weekend, when that CO was off base for R&R, and processed the orders through the stand-in CO. He was finally able to board a ship bound for home in December 1945, long after most of his fellow soldiers had returned to their families.

After coming back to the States in early 1946, Dad went on to finish his neurosurgical training with his friend and Harvard Medical School classmate, Donald Matson, who had served in the European Theater. They trained at the Peter Bent Brigham and the Children's Hospitals in Boston (flagship hospitals of Harvard Medical School) under Dr. Franc D. Ingraham, who had been one of the last residents trained by Dr. Harvey Cushing, globally regarded as the father of modern neurosurgery. In the 1950s and 1960s, the entire cadre of "3131C" neurosurgeons (as they were officially classified by the Army Air Force), who had honed their craft on the battlefields of Europe and the Pacific, went on to set the bar for the next half century of neurosurgeons, including those in my own generation.

My parents grew up during the Depression and were hardwired for work. Dad just about always made it home for family dinner at 7 P.M., usually in a suit and tie, but occasionally wearing surgical scrubs. Then he'd return to the hospital, often taking one of us kids along to do our homework in his office, while he made rounds on his patients. For Dad, life and work were essentially synonymous, and he raised us accordingly. He usually made my sisters and me do yard work on Sundays. If we told him we wanted to go to the movies, he'd reply: "If you go to the movies, then someone else has to work." He was also fiercely competitive. On the squash court, he considered every game a "battle to the death," and even into his eighties was always in search of fresh opponents, often decades younger.

He was a demanding parent, but also a wonderful one. He treated everyone he met with respect and carried a screwdriver in the pocket of his lab coat to tighten any loose screws he might encounter during his rounds of the hospital. His patients, his fellow physicians, the nurses, and the entire hospital staff loved him. Whether it was operating on patients, helping to advance research, training neurosurgeons (a singular passsion), or editing the journal *Surgical Neurology* (which he did for a number of years), Dad saw his path in life clearly marked out for him. Even after he finally aged out of the operating room at seventy-one, he continued to keep up with the latest developments in the field. After his death in 2004, his long-time partner Dr. David L. Kelly, Jr., wrote, "Dr. Alexander will always be remembered for his enthusiasm and proficiencies, his perseverance, and attention to detail, his spirit of compassion, honesty, and excellence in all that he did." No great surprise that I, like so many others, worshipped him.

Very early on, so far back I don't even remember when it was, Mom and Dad had told me that I was adopted (or "chosen," as they put it, because, they assured me, they'd known I was their child from the moment they saw me). They were not my biological birth parents, but they loved me dearly, as if I were their own flesh and blood. I grew up knowing that I'd been adopted in April 1954, at the age of four months, and that my biological mother had been sixteen years old—a sophomore in high school—unwed when she gave birth to me in 1953. Her boyfriend, a senior with no immediate prospects for being able to support a child, had agreed to give me up as well, though neither had wanted to. The knowledge of all this came so early that it was simply a part of who I was, as accepted and unquestioned as the jet black color of my hair and the fact that I liked hamburgers and disliked cauliflower. I loved my adoptive parents just as much as I would have if they had been true blood relations, and they clearly felt the same about me.

My older sister, Jean, had also been adopted, but five months after they adopted me, my mother was able to conceive herself. She delivered a baby girl—my sister Betsy—and five years later, Phyllis, our youngest sister, was born. We were full siblings for all intents and purposes. I knew that wherever I had come from, I was their brother and they were my sisters. I grew up in a family that not only loved me but also believed in me and supported my dreams. Including the dream that seized me in high school and never let go till I achieved it: to be a neurosurgeon like my father.

I didn't think about my adoption during my college and medical school years—at least not on the surface. I did reach out to the Children's Home Society of North Carolina several times, inquiring whether or not my mother had any interest in reuniting. But North Carolina had some of the nation's strictest laws to protect the anonymity of adoptees and their birth parents, even if they desperately wanted to reconnect. After my late twenties, I thought about the matter less and less. And once I met Holley and we started our own family, the question drifted ever further away.

Or ever deeper inside.

In 1999, when he was twelve and we were still living in Massachusetts, Eben IV got involved in a family heritage project at the Charles River School where he was a sixth grader. He knew I'd been adopted, and thus that he had direct relatives on the planet whom he didn't know personally, or even by name. The project sparked something in him—a deep curiosity that he hadn't, up to that point, known he had.

He asked me if we could seek out my birth parents. I told him that over the years I'd occasionally looked into the matter myself, contacting the Children's Home Society of North Carolina and asking if they had any news. If my biological mom or dad desired contact, the society would know. But I had never heard anything back.

Not that it bothered me. "It's perfectly natural in a circumstance like this," I'd told Eben. "It doesn't mean my birth mom doesn't love me, or that she wouldn't love you if she ever set eyes on you. But she doesn't want to, most likely because she feels like you and I have our own family and she doesn't want to get in the way of that."

Eben wouldn't let it go, though, so finally I thought I'd humor him and wrote a social worker named Betty at the Children's Home who'd helped me with my requests before. A few weeks later, on a snowy Friday afternoon in February 2000, Eben IV and I were driving from Boston up to Maine for a weekend of skiing when I remembered I was due to give Betty a call to check on her progress. I called her on my cell phone, and she answered.

"Well, in fact," she said, "I *do* have some news. Are you sitting down?"

I was in fact sitting down, so I said as much, omitting that I was also driving my car through a blizzard.

"It turns out, Dr. Alexander, that your birth parents actually *got married.*"

My heart hammered in my chest, and the road in front of me suddenly turned unreal and far away. Though I'd known that my parents were sweethearts, I'd always assumed that once they'd given me up, their lives had taken separate directions. Instantly a picture appeared in my head. A picture of my birth parents, and of a home that they'd made somewhere. A home I had never known. A home where—I didn't belong.

Betty interrupted my thoughts. "Dr. Alexander?"

"Yes," I said slowly, "I'm here."

"There's more."

To Eben's puzzlement, I pulled the car over to the side of the road and told her to go ahead.

"Your parents had three more children: Two sisters and a brother. I've been in touch with the older sister, and she told me your younger sister died two years ago. Your parents are still grieving their loss."

"So that means . . . ?" I asked after a long pause, still numb, taking it all in without really being able to process any of it.

"I'm sorry, Dr. Alexander, but yes—it means she is refusing your request for contact."

Eben shifted in the seat behind me, clearly aware that something of importance had just happened but stumped as to what it was.

"What is it, Dad?" he asked after I'd hung up.

"Nothing," I said. "The agency still doesn't know much, but they're working on it. Maybe some time later. Maybe . . ."

But my voice trailed off. Outside, the storm was really picking up. I could only see about a hundred yards into the low white woods spreading out all around us. I put the car in gear, squinted carefully into the rearview mirror, and pulled back onto the road.

In an instant, my view of myself had been totally changed. After that phone call I was, of course, still everything I'd been before: still a scientist, still a doctor, still a father, still a husband. But I also felt, for the first time ever, like an orphan. Someone who had been given away. Someone less than fully, 100 percent wanted.

I had never, before that phone call, really thought of myself that way—as someone cut off from my source. I'd never defined myself in the context of something I had lost and could never regain. But suddenly it was the only thing about myself I could see.

Over the next few months an ocean of sadness opened up within me: a sadness that threatened to swamp, and sink, everything in my life I'd worked so hard to create up to that point.

This was only made worse by my inability to get to the bottom of what was causing the situation. I'd run into problems in myself before—shortcomings, as I'd seen them—and I'd corrected them. In med school and in my early days as a surgeon, for example, I'd been part of a culture where heavy drinking, under the right circumstances, was smiled upon. But in 1991 I began to notice that I was looking forward to my day off, and the drinks that went along with it, just a little too eagerly. I decided that it was time for me to stop drinking alcohol altogether. This was not easy by any stretch—I'd come to rely on the release provided by those off hours more than I'd known—and I only made it through those early days of sobriety with my family's support. So here was another problem, clearly with only me to blame for it. I had help to deal with it if I chose to ask. Why couldn't I nip it in the bud? It just didn't seem right that a piece of knowledge about my past—a piece I had no control over whatsoever—should be able to so completely derail me both emotionally and professionally.

So I struggled. And I watched in disbelief as my roles as doctor, father, and husband became ever more difficult to fulfill. Seeing that I was not my best self, Holley set us up for a course of couples counseling. Though she only partially understood what was causing it, she forgave me for falling into this ditch of despair and did whatever she could to pull me up out of it. My depression had ramifications in my work. My parents were, of course, aware of this change, and though I knew they too forgave it, it killed me that my career in academic neurosurgery was slumping—and all they could do was watch from the sidelines. Without my participation, my family was powerless to help me.

And finally, I watched as this new sadness exposed, then swept away, something else: my last, half-acknowledged hope that there was some personal element in the universe—some force beyond the scientific ones I'd spent years studying. In less clinical terms, it swept away my last belief that there might be a Being of some kind out there who truly loved and cared about me—and that my prayers might be heard, and even answered. After that phone call during the blizzard, the notion of a loving, personal God—my birthright, to some degree, as a church-going member of a culture that took that God with genuine seriousness—vanished completely.

Was there a force or intelligence watching out for all of us?

Who cared about humans in a truly loving way? It was a surprise to have to finally admit that in spite of all my medical training and experience, I was clearly still keenly, if secretly, interested in this question, just as I'd been much more interested in the question of my birth parents than I'd ever realized.

Unfortunately, the answer to the question of whether there was such a Being was the same as the answer to the question of whether my birth parents would once again open their lives and their hearts to me.

That answer was no.

11

An End to the Downward Spiral

For much of the next seven years my career, and my family life, continued to suffer. For a long time the people around me—even those closest to me—weren't sure what was causing the problem. But gradually—through remarks I'd make almost in passing—Holley and my sisters put the pieces together.

Finally, on an early morning walk on a South Carolina beach during a family vacation in July 2007, Betsy and Phyllis brought up the topic. "Have you thought about writing another letter to your birth family?" Phyllis asked.

"Yes," Betsy said. "Things might have changed by now, you never know." Betsy had recently told us she was thinking of adopting a child herself, so I wasn't totally surprised that the topic had come up. But all the same, my immediate response—mental rather than verbal—was: *Oh no, not again!* I remembered the immense chasm that had cracked open beneath me after the rejection I'd faced seven years earlier. But I knew Betsy and Phyllis's hearts were in the right place. They knew I was suffering, they'd finally figured out why, and they wanted—rightly—for me to step up and try to fix the problem. They assured me that they would travel this road with me—that I wouldn't be taking this journey alone, as I had done before. We were a team.

So in early August 2007, I wrote an anonymous letter to my birth sister, the keeper of the gate on the matter, and sent it to Betty at the Children's Home Society of North Carolina to forward along:

Dear Sister,

I am interested in communicating with you, our brother and our parents. After a long talk with my adoptive family sisters and mother about this, their support and interest rekindled my wanting to know more about my biological family.

My two sons, ages 9 and 19, are interested in their heritage. The three of us and my wife would be grateful to you for any background information that you feel comfortable sharing. For me, questions come to mind about my birth parents regarding their lives in their younger years until now. What interests and personalities do you all have?

In that we are all growing older, my hopes are to meet them soon. Our arrangements can be in mutual agreement. Please know that I feel most respectful of the degree of privacy that they wish to maintain. I have had a wonderful adoptive family and appreciate my biological parents' decision in their youth. My interest is genuine and receptive to any boundaries they feel are necessary.

Your consideration in this matter is deeply appreciated.

Most sincerely yours,
Your older Brother

A few weeks later I received a letter from the Children's Home Society. It was from my birth sister.

"Yes, we would love to meet you," she wrote. North Carolina state law forbade her from revealing any identifying information to me, but working around those parameters, she gave me my first real set of clues about the biological family I had never met.

When she reported that my birth father had been a naval

aviator in Vietnam, it just blew me away: no wonder I had always loved to jump out of airplanes and fly sailplanes. My birth dad was also, I was further stunned to learn, an astronaut trainee with NASA during the Apollo missions in the mid-1960s (I myself had considered training as a mission specialist on the space shuttle in 1983). My birth dad later worked as an airline pilot for Pan Am and Delta.

In October 2007, I finally met my biological parents, Ann and Richard, and my biological siblings, Kathy and David. Ann told me the full story of how, in 1953, she spent three months at the Florence Crittenden Home for Unwed Mothers, located next to Charlotte Memorial Hospital. All of the girls there had code names, and because she loved American history, my mother chose Virginia Dare—the name of the first baby born to English settlers in the New World. Most of the girls just called her Dare. At sixteen, she was the youngest girl there.

She told me that her daddy had been willing to do anything to help her when he learned of her "predicament." He was willing to pick up and move the whole family if necessary. He had been unemployed for a while, and bringing a new baby into the home would be a great financial stress, not to mention all the other problems.

A close friend of his had even mentioned a doctor he knew of down in Dillon, South Carolina, who could "fix things." But her mother wouldn't hear of *that*.

Ann told me how she had looked up at the stars twinkling wildly in the gusty winds of a newly arrived cold front on that frigid December night in 1953—how she had walked across the empty streets under scattered low, racing clouds. She had wanted this time to be alone, with just the moon and stars and her soon-to-be-born child—me.

"The crescent moon hung low in the west. Brilliant Jupiter was just rising, to watch over us all night. Richard loved science and astronomy, and he later told me that Jupiter was at opposition that night, and would not be as bright again for almost nine years. Over that time, much would happen in our lives, including the births of two more children.

"But at the time I just thought how beautiful and bright the King of Planets appeared, watching over us from above."

As she entered the hospital foyer, a magical thought struck her. Girls generally stayed in the Crittenden Home for two weeks after they delivered their babies, then they'd go home and pick up their lives where they'd left off. If she really delivered that night, she and I might be home for Christmas—if they actually set her free at two weeks. What a perfect miracle that would be: to bring me home by Christmas Day.

"Dr. Crawford was fresh from another delivery, and he looked awfully tired," Ann told me. He laid an ether-soaked gauze over her face to ease the pain, so she was only semiconscious when finally, at 2:42 A.M., with one last great push, she gave birth to her first child.

Ann told me that she wanted so much to hold and caress me, and that she would never forget hearing my cries until fatigue and that anesthetic finally won out.

Over the next four hours, first Mars, then Saturn, then Mercury, and finally brilliant Venus rose in the eastern sky to greet me into this world. Meanwhile, Ann slept more deeply than she had in months.

The nurse awakened her before sunrise.

"I have someone I want you to meet," she said cheerfully, and presented me, swaddled in a sky-blue blanket, for her to admire.

"The nurses all agreed that you were the most beautiful baby in the whole nursery. I was bursting with pride."

As much as Ann wanted to keep me, the cold reality that she couldn't soon sank in. Richard had dreams of going to college, but those dreams would not keep me fed. Perhaps I felt Ann's pain, because I stopped eating. At eleven days, I was hospitalized with the diagnosis that I was "failing to thrive," and my first Christmas and the following nine days were spent in the hospital in Charlotte.

After I was admitted to the hospital, Ann took the two-hour bus ride north to her small hometown. She spent that Christmas with her parents, sisters, and friends, whom she had not seen in three months. All without me.

By the time I was eating again, my separate life was under way. Ann sensed that she was losing control and that they weren't going to allow her to keep me. When she called the hospital just after New Year's, she was told that I had been sent to the Children's Home Society in Greensboro.

"Sent with a volunteer? How unfair!" she said.

I spent the next three months living in a baby dorm with several other infants whose mothers could not keep them. My crib was on the second floor of a bluish gray Victorian home that had been donated to the society. "It was a most pleasant place for your first home," Ann told me with a laugh, "even though it was mainly a baby dorm." Ann took the three-hour bus ride to visit half a dozen times over the next few months, trying desperately to come up with a plan that would succeed in keeping me with her. Once she came with her mother and another time with Richard (although the nurses made him view me through the window—they would not let him in the same room, and certainly not let him hold me).

But by late March 1954, it was clear that things weren't going to go her way. She would have to give me up. She and her mother took the bus to Greensboro one last time.

"I had to hold you and look in your eyes and try to explain it all to you," Ann told me. "I knew you would just giggle and coo, blow baby bubbles, and make pleasing sounds no matter what I said, but I felt I owed you an explanation. I held you closely one last time, kissed your ears, chest, and face, and caressed you gently. I remember inhaling deeply, loving that wonderful aroma of freshly bathed baby, as if it were yesterday.

"I called you by your birth name and said, 'I love you so much, so much you'll never know. And I'll love you forever, until the day I die.'

"I said, 'God, please let him know how much he is loved. That I love him, and always will.' But I had no way of knowing if my prayer would be answered. Adoption arrangements in the 1950s were final and very secret. No turning back, no explanations. Sometimes birth dates were changed in the records just to hamper anyone's efforts to uncover the truth about a baby's origins. Leave nothing to trace. Agreements were protected by harsh state laws. The rule was to forget it ever happened and go on with the rest of your life. And, hopefully, learn from it.

"I kissed you one last time, then laid you gently in your crib. I wrapped you in your little blue blanket, took one last look into your blue eyes, then kissed my finger and touched it to your forehead.

" 'Goodbye, Richard Michael. I love you,' were my last words to you, at least for half a century or so."

Ann went on to tell me that after she and Richard were married and the rest of their children came along, she became more and more taken up with finding out what had become of me. In addition to being a naval aviator and an airline pilot, Richard was an attorney, and Ann figured that gave him license to uncover my adoptive identity. But Richard was too much of a gentleman to go back on the adoption agreement made in 1954, and he kept out of the matter. In the early 1970s, with the war in Vietnam still raging, Ann couldn't get the date of my birth out of her head. I would turn nineteen in December 1972. Would I go over? If so, what would become of me there? Early on, my plan was to enlist in the marines to fly. My vision was 20/100, and the Air Force required 20/20 without correction. Word on the street was that the marines would take even those of us with 20/100 vision and teach us to fly. However, they then started winding down the Vietnam war effort, so I never enlisted. I headed off to med school instead. But Ann knew none of this. In the spring of 1973, they watched as surviving POWs from the "Hanoi Hilton" disembarked from the planes returning from North Vietnam. They were heartbroken when missing pilots they knew, more than half of Richard's navy class, failed to emerge from the planes, and Ann got it in her head that I might have been killed over there myself.

Once in her mind the image refused to fade, and for years she was convinced that I'd died a grisly death in the rice paddies of Vietnam. She certainly would have been surprised to know that at that time I was just a few miles away from her in Chapel Hill!

In the summer of 2008, I met up with my biological father, his brother Bob, and his brother-in-law, also named Bob, at Litchfield Beach, South Carolina. Brother Bob was a decorated hero in the navy during the Korean War and a test pilot at China Lake (the navy's weapons test center in the California desert, where he perfected the Sidewinder missile system and flew F-104 Starfighters). Meanwhile Richard's brother-in-law Bob set a speed record during Operation Sun Run in 1957, a circumglobal relay record in F-101 Voodoo jet fighters "outflying the sun" by circling the earth at an average speed of over 1,000 miles per hour.

It felt like Old Home Week for me.

Those meetings with my birth parents heralded the end of what I've come to think of as my Years of Not Knowing. Years that, I came at last to learn, had been characterized by the same terrible pain for my birthparents as they had been for me.

There was only one wound that wouldn't heal: the loss, ten years earlier in 1998, of my biological sister Betsy (yes, the same name as one of the sisters in my adoptive family, and they both married Robs, but that's another story). She'd had a big heart, everyone told me, and, when not working at the rape crisis center where she spent most of her time, she could usually be found feeding and caring for a menagerie of stray dogs and cats. "A real angel," Ann called her. Kathy promised to send me a picture of her. Betsy had struggled with alcohol just as I had, and learning of her loss, fueled in part by those struggles, made me realize once again how fortunate I had been in resolving my own problem. I longed to meet Betsy, to comfort her—to tell her that wounds could heal, and that all would be okay.

Because, strangely enough, meeting my birth family was the first time in my life that I felt that things really *were*, somehow, okay. Family mattered, and I'd gotten mine—most of mine— back. This was my first real education in how profoundly knowledge of one's origins can heal a person's life in unexpected ways.

Knowing where I came from, my biological origins, allowed me to see, and to accept, things in myself that I'd never dreamed I'd have been able to. Through meeting them, I was allowed to throw away, at last, the nagging suspicion that I'd carried around without even being aware of it: a suspicion that, wherever I *had* come from, biologically speaking, I had not been loved or cared about. Subconsciously, I had believed that I *didn't deserve* to be loved, or even to exist. Discovering that I had been loved, since the very beginning, began to heal me in the most profound way imaginable. I felt a wholeness I had never known before.

It was not, however, the only discovery in this area that I would make. The other question that I thought had been answered in the car with Eben that day—the question of whether there really is a loving God out there—still held, and the answer in my mind was still no.

It wasn't until I spent seven days in coma that I revisited that question. I discovered an entirely unexpected answer there as well . . .

The Core

Something pulled at me. Not like someone grabbing my arm, but something subtler, less physical. It was a little like when the sun dips behind a cloud and you feel your mood change instantly in response.

I was going back, away from the Core. Its inky-bright darkness faded into the green landscape of the Gateway, with all of its dazzling landscape. Looking down, I saw the villagers again, the trees and sparkling streams and the waterfalls, as well as the arcing angel-beings above.

My companion was there, too. She had been there the whole time, of course, all through my journey into the Core, in the form of that orblike ball of light. But now she was, once again, in human form. She wore the same beautiful dress, and seeing her again made me feel like a child lost in a huge and alien city who suddenly comes upon a familiar face. What a gift she was! "We will show you many things, but you will be going back." That message, delivered wordlessly to me at the entrance to the trackless darkness of the Core, came back to me now. I also now understood where "back" was.

The Realm of the Earthworm's-Eye View where I had started this odyssey.

But it was different this time. Moving down into the darkness with the full knowledge of what lay above it, I no longer experienced the trepidation that I had when I was originally there. As the glorious music of the Gateway faded out and the pulse-like pounding of the lower realm returned, I heard and saw these things as an adult sees a place where he or she had once been frightened but is no longer afraid. The murk and darkness, the faces that bubbled up and faded away, the artery-like roots that came down from above, held no terror for me now, because I understood—in the wordless way I understood everything then—that I was no longer *of* this place, but only visiting it.

But *why* was I visiting it again?

The answer came to me in the same instantaneous, nonverbal way that the answers in the brilliant world above had been delivered. This whole adventure, it began to occur to me, was some kind of tour—some kind of grand overview of the invisible, spiritual side of existence. And like all good tours, it included all floors and all levels.

Once I was back in the lower realm, the vagaries of time in these worlds beyond what I knew of this earth continued to hold. To get a little—if only a very little—idea of what this feels like, ponder how time lays itself out in dreams. In a dream, "before" and "after" become tricky designations. You can be in one part of the dream and know what's coming, even if you haven't experienced it yet. My "time" out beyond was something like that—though I should also underline that what happened to me had none of the murky confusion of our earthbound dreams, except at the very earliest stages, when I was still in the underworld.

How long was I there this time? Again I have no real idea—no way to gauge it. But I do know that after returning to the lower realm, it took a long time to discover that I actually had some control over my course—that I was no longer trapped in this lower world. With concerted effort, I could move back up to the higher planes. At a certain point in the murky depths,

I found myself wishing for the Spinning Melody to return. After an initial struggle to recall the notes, the gorgeous music, and the spinning ball of light emitting it blossomed into my awareness. They cut, once again, through the jellied muck, and I began to rise.

In the worlds above, I slowly discovered, to know and be able to think of something is all one needs in order to move toward it. To think of the Spinning Melody was to make it appear, and to long for the higher worlds was to bring myself there. The more familiar I became with the world above, the easier it was to return to it. During my time out of my body, I accomplished this back-and-forth movement from the muddy darkness of the Realm of the Earthworm's-Eye View to the green brilliance of the Gateway and into the black but holy darkness of the Core any number of times. How many I can't say exactly—again because time as it was there just doesn't translate to our conception of time here on earth. But each time I reached the Core, I went deeper than before, and was taught more, in the wordless, more-than-verbal way that all things are communicated in the worlds above this one.

That doesn't mean that I saw anything like the whole universe, either in my original journey from the Earthworm's-Eye View up to the Core, or in the ones that came afterward. In fact, one of the truths driven home to me in the Core each time I returned to it was how impossible it would be to understand all that exists—either its physical/visible side or its (much, much larger) spiritual/invisible side, not to mention the countless other universes that exist or have ever existed.

But none of that mattered, because I had already been taught the one thing—the only thing—that, in the last analysis, truly matters. I had initially received this piece of knowledge from my lovely companion on the butterfly wing upon my first entrance into the Gateway. It came in three parts, and to take one more shot at putting it into words (because of course it was initially delivered wordlessly), it would run something like this:

You are loved and cherished.

You have nothing to fear.

There is nothing you can do wrong.

If I had to boil this entire message down to one sentence, it would run this way:

You are loved.

And if I had to boil it down further, to just one word, it would (of course) be, simply:

Love.

Love is, without a doubt, the basis of everything. Not some abstract, hard-to-fathom kind of love but the day-to-day kind that everyone knows—the kind of love we feel when we look at our spouse and our children, or even our animals. In its purest and most powerful form, this love is not jealous or selfish, but *unconditional*. This is the reality of realities, the incomprehensibly glorious truth of truths that lives and breathes at the core of everything that exists or that ever will exist, and no remotely accurate understanding of who and what we are can be achieved by anyone who does not know it, and embody it in all of their actions.

Not much of a scientific insight? Well, I beg to differ. I'm back from that place, and nothing could convince me that this is not only the single most important emotional truth in the universe, but also the single most important *scientific* truth as well.

I've been talking about my experience, as well as meeting other people who study or have undergone near-death experiences, for several years now. I know that the term *unconditional love* gets bandied around a lot in those circles. How many of us can grasp what that truly means?

I know, of course, why the term comes up as much as it does. It's because many, many other people have seen and experienced what I did. But like me, when these people come back to the earthly level, they're stuck with words, and words alone, to convey experiences and insights that lie completely beyond the power of words. It's like trying to write a novel with only half the alphabet.

The primary hurdle that most NDE subjects must jump is not how to reacclimate to the limitations of the earthly world—though this can certainly be a challenge—but how to convey what the love they experienced out there *actually feels like.*

Deep down, we already know. Just as Dorothy in *The Wizard of Oz* always had the capability to return home, we have the ability to recover our connection with that idyllic realm. We just forget that we do, because during the brain-based, physical portion of our existence, our brain blocks out, or veils, that larger cosmic background, just as the sun's light blocks the stars from view each morning. Imagine how limited our view of the universe would be if we never saw the star-spangled nighttime sky.

We can only see what our brain's filter allows through. The brain—in particular its left-side linguistic/logical part, that which generates our sense of rationality and the feeling of being a sharply defined ego or self—is a barrier to our higher knowledge and experience.

It is my belief that we are now facing a crucial time in our existence. We need to recover more of that larger knowledge *while living here on earth,* while our brains (including its left-side analytical parts) are fully functioning. Science—the science to which I've devoted so much of my life—doesn't contradict what I learned up there. But far, far too many people believe it does, because certain members of the scientific community, who are pledged to the materialist worldview, have insisted again and again that science and spirituality cannot coexist.

They are mistaken. Making this ancient but ultimately basic fact more widely known is why I have written this book, and it renders all the other aspects of my story—the mystery of how I contracted my illness, of how I managed to be conscious in another dimension for the week of my coma, and how I somehow recovered so completely—entirely secondary.

The unconditional love and acceptance that I experienced on my journey is the single most important discovery I have ever made, or will ever make, and as hard as I know it's going to be to unpack the other lessons I learned while there, I also know in my heart that sharing this very basic message—one so simple that most children readily accept it—is the most important task I have.

13.

Wednesday

For two days, "Wednesday" had been the buzzword—the day on my doctors' lips when it came to describing my chances. As in: "We hope to see some improvement by Wednesday." And now here Wednesday was, without so much as a glimmer of change in my condition.

"When can I see Dad?"

This question—the natural one for a ten-year-old whose father is in the hospital—had been coming from Bond regularly since I had gone into a coma on Monday. Holley had been fending it off successfully for two days, but on Wednesday morning, she decided it was time to address it.

When Holley had told Bond, on Monday night, that I wasn't home from the hospital yet because I was "sick," he conjured what that word had always meant to him, up to this point in his ten years of life: a cough, a sore throat—maybe a headache. Granted, his appreciation of just how much a headache can actually hurt had been greatly expanded by what he'd seen on Monday morning. But when Holley finally brought him to the hospital that Wednesday afternoon, he was still hoping to be greeted by something very different from what he saw in my hospital bed.

Bond saw a body that already bore only a distant resemblance to what he knew as his father. When someone is sleeping, you can look at them and tell there's still a person inhabiting the body. There's a presence. But most doctors will tell you it's different when a person is in a coma (even if they can't tell you exactly why). The body is there, but there's a strange, almost physical sensation that the person is missing. That their essence, inexplicably, is somewhere else.

Eben IV and Bond had always been very close, ever since Eben ran into the delivery suite when Bond was only minutes old to hug his brand new brother. Eben met Bond at the hospital that third day of my coma and did what he could to frame the situation positively for his younger brother. And, being hardly more than a boy himself, he came up with a scenario he thought Bond would be able to appreciate: a battle.

"Let's make a picture of what's going on so Dad will see it when he gets better," he said to Bond.

So on a table in the hospital dining area, they laid out a big sheet of orange paper and drew a representation of what was happening inside my comatose body. They drew my white blood cells, wearing capes and armed with swords, defending the besieged territory of my brain. And, armed with their own swords and slightly different uniforms, they drew the invading *E. coli*. There was hand-to-hand combat, and the bodies of the slain on both sides were scattered about.

It was an accurate enough representation, in its way. The only thing about it that was inaccurate, taking into account the simplification of the obviously more complex event going on inside my body, was the way the battle was going. In Eben and Bond's rendition, the battle was pitched and at a white heat, with both sides struggling and the outcome uncertain—though, of course, the white blood cells would eventually win. But as he sat with Bond, colored markers spread out on the table, trying to share in this naïve version of events, Eben knew that in truth, the battle was no longer pitched, or so uncertain.

And he knew which side was winning.

14

A Special Kind of NDE

The true value of a human being is determined primarily by the measure and the sense in which he has attained liberation from the self.

—ALBERT EINSTEIN (1879–1955)

W hen I was initially in the Realm of the Earthworm's-Eye View, I had no real center of consciousness. I didn't know who or what I was, or even *if* I was. I was simply . . . *there*, a singular awareness in the midst of a soupy, dark, muddy nothingness that had no beginning and, seemingly, no end.

Now, however, I knew. I understood that I was part of the Divine and that nothing—absolutely nothing—could ever take that away. The (false) suspicion that we can somehow be separated from God is the root of every form of anxiety in the universe, and the cure for it—which I received partially within the Gateway and completely within the Core—was the knowledge that nothing can tear us from God, ever. This knowledge—and it remains the single most important thing I've ever learned—robbed the Realm of the Earthworm's-Eye View of its terror and allowed me to see it for what it really was: a not entirely pleasant, but no doubt necessary, part of the cosmos.

Many people have traveled to the realms I did, but, strangely enough, most remembered their earthly identities while away from their earthly forms. They knew that they were John Smith or George Johnson or Sarah Brown. They never lost sight of the fact that they lived on earth. They were aware that their living relatives were still there, waiting and hoping they would come back. They also, in many cases, met friends and relatives who had died before them, and in these cases, too, they recognized those people instantly.

Many NDE subjects have reported engaging in life reviews, in which they saw their interactions with various people and their good or bad actions during the course of their lives.

I experienced none of these events, and taken all together they demonstrate the single most unusual aspect of my NDE. I was completely free of my bodily identity for all of it, so that any classic NDE occurrence that might have involved my re-membering who I was on earth was rigorously missing.

To say that at that point in the proceedings I still had no idea who I was or where I'd come from sounds somewhat perplexing, I know. After all, how could I be learning all these stunningly complex and beautiful things, how could I see the girl next to me, and the blossoming trees and waterfalls and villagers, and still not know that it was I, Eben Alexander, who was the one experiencing them? How could I understand all that I did, yet not realize that on earth I was a doctor, husband, and father? A person who was not seeing trees and rivers and clouds for the first time when I entered the Gateway, but one who had seen more than his share of them as a child growing up in the very concrete and earthly locale of Winston-Salem, North Carolina?

My best shot at an answer is to suggest that I was in a position similar to that of someone with partial but beneficial amnesia. That is, a person *who has forgotten some key aspect about him or herself,* but *who benefits through having forgotten it,* even if for only a short while.

How did I gain from not remembering my earthly self? It allowed me to go deep into realms beyond the worldly without having to worry about what I was leaving behind. Throughout my entire time in those worlds, I was a soul with nothing to lose. No places to miss, no people to mourn. I had come from nowhere and had no history, so I fully accepted my circumstances—even the initial murk and mess of the Realm of the Earthworm's-Eye View—with equanimity.

And because I so completely forgot my mortal identity, I was granted full access to the true cosmic being I really am (and *we* all are). Once again, in some ways my experience was analogous to a dream, in which you remember some things about yourself while forgetting other things completely. But again this is only a partially useful analogy, because, as I keep stressing, the Gateway and the Core were not remotely dreamlike but ultra-real—as far from illusory as one can be. To use the word *removed* makes it sound as if the absence of my earthly memories while in the Realm of the Earthworm's-Eye View, the Gateway, and the Core was in some manner intentional. I now suspect that this was the case. At the risk of oversimplifying, I was allowed to die harder, and travel deeper, than almost all NDE subjects before me.

As arrogant as that might sound, my intentions are not. The rich literature on NDEs has proved crucial to understanding my own journey in coma. I can't claim to know why I had the experience I had, but I do know now (three years later), from reading other NDE literature, that the penetration of the higher worlds tends to be a gradual process and requires that the individual release his or her attachments to whatever level he or she is on before going higher or deeper.

That was not a problem for me, because throughout my experience I had no earthly memories whatsoever, and the only pain and heartache I felt was when I had to return to earth, where I'd begun.

15

The Gift of Forgetting

We must believe in free will. We have no choice.

—Isaac B. Singer (1902–1991)

The view of human consciousness held by most scientists today is that it is composed of digital information—data, that is, of essentially the same kind used by computers. Though some bits of this data—seeing a spectacular sunset, hearing a beautiful symphony for the first time, even falling in love—may feel more profound or special to us than the countless other bits of information created and stored in our brains, this is really just an illusion. All bits are, in fact, qualitatively the same. Our brains model outside reality by taking the information that comes in through our senses and transforming it into a rich digital tapestry. But our perceptions are just a model—not reality itself. An *illusion*.

This was, of course, the view I held as well. I can remember being in medical school and occasionally hearing arguments that consciousness is nothing more than a very complex computer program. These arguments suggested that the ten billion or so neurons firing constantly within our brains are capable of producing a lifetime of consciousness and memory.

To understand how the brain might actually block our access to knowledge of the higher worlds, we need to accept—at least hypothetically and for the moment—that the brain itself doesn't produce consciousness. That it is, instead, a kind of reducing valve or filter, shifting the larger, nonphysical consciousness that we possess in the nonphysical worlds down into a more limited capacity for the duration of our mortal lives. There is, from the earthly perspective, a very definite advantage to this. Just as our brains work hard every moment of our waking lives to filter out the barrage of sensory information coming at us from our physical surroundings, selecting the material we actually need in order to survive, so it is that forgetting our trans-earthly identities also allows us to be "here and now" far more effectively. Just as most of ordinary life holds too much information for us to take in at once and still get anything done, being excessively conscious of the worlds beyond the here and now would slow down our progress even more. If we knew too much of the spiritual realm now, then navigating our lives on earth would be an even greater challenge than it already is. (That's not to say we shouldn't be conscious of the worlds beyond now—only that if we are extra-conscious of their grandeur and immensity, they can prevent action while still here on earth.) From a more purpose-focused perspective (and I now believe the universe is nothing if not purposeful), making the right decisions through our free will in the face of the evil and injustice on earth would mean far less if we remembered, while here, the full beauty and brilliance of what awaits us.

Why am I so sure of all this? For two reasons. The first is that I was shown it (by the beings who taught me when I was in the Gateway and the Core), and the second is because I actually experienced it. While beyond my body, I received knowledge about the nature and structure of the universe that was vastly beyond my comprehension. But I received it anyhow, in large part because, with my worldly preoccupations out of the way, I had room to do so. Now that I'm back on earth and remember my bodily identity, the seed of that trans-earthly knowledge has once again been covered over. And yet it's still there. I can feel it, at every moment. It will take years, in this earthly environment, to come to fruition. That is, it will take me years to understand, using my mortal, material brain, what I understood so instantly and easily in the brain-free realms of the world beyond. Yet I'm confident that with hard work on my part, much of that knowledge will continue to unfold.

To say that there is still a chasm between our current scientific understanding of the universe and the truth as I saw it is a considerable understatement. I still love physics and cosmology, still love studying our vast and wonderful universe. Only I now have a greatly enlarged conception of what "vast" and "wonderful" really mean. The physical side of the universe is as a speck of dust compared to the invisible and spiritual part. In my past view, *spiritual* wasn't a word that I would have employed during a scientific conversation. Now I believe it is a word that we cannot afford to leave out.

From the Core, my understanding of what we call "dark energy" and "dark matter" seemed to have clear explanations, as did far more advanced components of the makeup of our universe that humans won't address for ages.

This doesn't mean, however, that I can explain them to you. That's because—paradoxically—I am still in the process of understanding them myself. Perhaps the best way of conveying that part of the experience is to say that I had a foretaste of another, larger kind of knowledge: one I believe human beings will be able to access in ever larger numbers in the future. But conveying that knowledge now is rather like being a chimpanzee, becoming a human for a single day to experience all of the wonders of human knowledge, and then returning to one's chimp friends and trying to tell them what it was like knowing several different Romance languages, the calculus, and the immense scale of the universe.

Up there, a question would arise in my mind, and the answer would arise at the same time, like a flower coming up right next to it. It was almost as if, just as no physical particle in the universe is really separate from another, so in the same way there was no such thing as a question without an accompanying answer. These answers were not simple "yes" or "no" fare, either. They were vast conceptual edifices, staggering structures of living thought, as intricate as cities. Ideas so vast they would have taken me lifetimes to find my way around it I had been confined to earthly thought. But I wasn't. I had sloughed off that earthly style of thought like a butterfly breaking from a chrysalis.

I saw the earth as a pale blue dot in the immense blackness of physical space. I could see that earth was a place where good and evil mixed, and that this constituted one of its unique features. Even on earth there is much more good than evil, but earth is a place where evil is allowed to gain influence in a way that would be entirely impossible at higher levels of existence. That evil could occasionally have the upper hand was known and allowed by the Creator as a necessary consequence of giving the gift of free will to beings like us.

Small particles of evil were scattered throughout the universe, but the sum total of all that evil was as a grain of sand on a vast beach compared to the goodness, abundance, hope, and unconditional love in which the universe was literally awash. The very fabric of the alternate dimension is love and acceptance, and anything that does not have these qualities appears immediately and obviously out of place there.

But free will comes at the cost of a loss or falling-away from this love and acceptance. We are free; but we are free beings hemmed all around by an environment conspiring to make us feel that we are not free. Free will is of central importance for our function in the earthly realm: a function that, we will all one day discover, serves the much higher role of allowing our ascendance in the timeless alternate dimension. Our life down here may seem insignificant, for it is minute in relation to the other lives and other worlds that also crowd the invisible and visible universes. But it is also hugely important, for our role here is to grow toward the Divine, and that growth is closely watched by the beings in the worlds above—the souls and lucent orbs (those beings I saw originally far above me in the Gateway, and which I believe are the origin of our culture's concept of angels).

We—the spiritual beings currently inhabiting our evolutionarily developed mortal brains and bodies, the product of the earth and the exigencies of the earth—make the real choices. True thought is not the brain's affair. But we have—in part by the brain itself—been so trained to associate our brains with what we think and who we are that we have lost the ability to realize that we are at all times much more than the physical brains and bodies that do—or should do—our bidding.

True thought is pre-physical. This is the thinking-behind-the-thinking responsible for all the genuinely consequential choices we make in the world. A thinking that is not dependent on linear deduction, but that moves fast as lightning, making connections on different levels, bringing them together. In the face of this free, inner intelligence, our ordinary thought is hopelessly slow and fumbling. It's this thinking that catches the football in the end zone, that comes up with the inspired scientific insight or writes the inspired song. The subliminal thinking that is always there, when we really need it, but that we have all too often lost the ability both to access and to believe in. Needless to say, it's the thinking that sprang into action the evening of that skydive when Chuck's chute opened up suddenly beneath me.

To experience thinking outside the brain is to enter a world of instantaneous connections that make ordinary thinking (i.e., those aspects limited by the physical brain and the speed of light) seem like some hopelessly sleepy and plodding event. Our truest, deepest self is completely free. It is not crippled or compromised by past actions or concerned with identity or status. It comprehends that it has no need to fear the earthly world, and therefore, it has no need to build itself up through fame or wealth or conquest.

This is the true spiritual self that all of us are destined someday to recover. But until that day comes, I feel, we should do everything in our power to get in touch with this miraculous aspect of ourselves—to cultivate it and bring it to light. This is the being living within all of us right now and that is, in fact, the being that God truly intends us to be.

How do we get closer to this genuine spiritual self? By manifesting love and compassion. Why? Because love and compassion are far more than the abstractions many of us believe them to be. They are real. They are concrete. And they make up the very fabric of the spiritual realm.

In order to return to that realm, we must once again become *like* that realm, even while we are stuck in, and plodding through, this one.

One of the biggest mistakes people make when they think about God is to imagine God as impersonal. Yes, God is behind the numbers, the perfection of the universe that science measures and struggles to understand. But—again, paradoxically—Om is "human" as well—even *more* human than you and I are. Om understands and sympathizes with our human situation more profoundly and personally than we can even imagine because Om knows what we have forgotten, and understands the terrible burden it is to live with amnesia of the Divine for even a moment.

16

The Well

Holley first met our friend Sylvia in the 1980s, when both were teaching at the Ravenscroft School in Raleigh, North Carolina. While there, Holley was also a close friend of Susan Reintjes. Susan is an intuitive—a fact that never got in the way of my feelings about her. She was, to my mind, a very special person, even if what she did was, to say the least, outside my straight-and-narrow neurosurgical view. She was also a channel and had written a book called *Third Eye Open,* which Holley was a big fan of. One of the spiritual healing activities Susan regularly performed involved helping coma patients to heal by contacting them psychically. On Thursday, my fourth day in coma, Sylvia had the idea that Susan should try to contact me.

Sylvia called her at home in Chapel Hill and explained what was happening with me. Would it be possible for her to "tune in" to me? Susan said yes and asked for a few details about my illness. Sylvia gave her the basics: I'd been in a coma for four days and I was in critical condition.

"That's all I need to know," Susan said. "I'll try to contact him tonight."

According to Susan's view, a coma patient was a kind of in-between being. Neither completely here (the earthly realm) nor completely there (the spiritual realm), these patients often have a singularly mysterious atmosphere to them. This was, as I've mentioned, a phenomenon I'd noticed myself many times, though of course I'd never given it the supernatural credence that Susan had.

In Susan's experience, one of the qualities that set coma patients apart was their receptivity to telepathic communication. She was confident that once she'd put herself into a meditative state, she'd soon establish contact with me.

"Communicating with a coma patient," she later told me, "is a little like throwing a rope down a deep well. How deep the rope needs to go depends on the depth of the comatose state. When I tried to contact you, the first thing that surprised me was how deep the rope went. The farther down, the more frightened I became that you were too far away—that I wouldn't be able to reach you because you weren't coming back."

After five full minutes of mentally descending via the telepathic "rope," she felt a slight shift, like a fishing line deep down in the water getting a small but definite tug.

"I was sure it was you," she told me later, "and I told Holley as much. I told her it wasn't your time yet, and that your body would know what to do. I suggested that Holley keep those two thoughts in mind, and repeat them to you at your bedside."

17

N of 1

It was Thursday when my doctors determined that my particular strain of E. *coli* didn't match the ultraresistant strain that, unaccountably, had shown up in Israel just at the time I'd been there. But the fact that it didn't match only made my case more confounding. While it was certainly good news that I was not harboring a strain of bacteria that could wipe out a third of the country, in terms of my own, individual recovery, it just underscored what my doctors were already suspecting all too clearly: that my case was essentially without precedent.

It was also quickly moving from desperate to hopeless. The doctors simply didn't have an answer for how I could have contracted my illness, or how I could be brought back from my coma. They were sure of only one thing: they did not know of anyone making a full recovery from bacterial meningitis after being comatose for more than a few days. We were now into day four.

The stress took its toll on everyone. Phyllis and Betsy had decided on Tuesday that any talk of the possibility of my dying would be forbidden in my presence, under the assumption that some part of me might be aware of the discussion. Early Thursday morning, Jean asked one of the nurses in the ICU room about my chances of survival. Betsy, on the other side of my bed, heard her and said: "*Please* don't have that conversation in this room."

Jean and I had always been extremely close. We were part of

the family just like our "homegrown" siblings, but the fact that we were "chosen" by mom and dad, as they put it, inevitably gave us a special bond. She had always watched out for me, and her frustration at her powerlessness over the current situation brought her close to a breaking point.

Tears came to Jean's eyes. "I need to go home for a while," she said.

After determining that there were plenty of people to continue my bedside vigil, all agreed that the nursing staff would probably be delighted to have one less person in my room.

Jean went back to our home, packed her bags, and drove home to Delaware that afternoon. By leaving, she gave the first real outward expression to an emotion the whole family was starting to feel: powerlessness. There are few experiences more frustrating than seeing a loved one in a comatose state. You want to help, but you can't. You want the person to open his or her eyes, but they don't. Families of coma patients often resort to opening the patient's eyes themselves. It's a way of forcing the issue—of ordering the patient to wake up. Of course it doesn't work, and it can also further damage morale. Patients in deep coma lose the coordination of their eyes and pupils. Open the lids of a deep coma patient, and you're likely to find one eye pointing in one direction, the other in the opposite. It's an unnerving sight, and it added further to Holley's pain several times that week when she pried my eyelids open and saw, in essence, the askew eyeballs of a corpse.

With Jean gone, things really started to fray. Phyllis now began to exhibit a behavior I'd also seen countless times among patients' family members in my own practice. She started to become frustrated with my doctors.

"Why aren't they giving us more information?" she asked

Betsy, outraged. "I swear, if Eben were here, *he* would tell us what's really going on."

The fact was that my doctors were doing absolutely everything they could do for me. Phyllis, of course, knew this. But the pain and frustration of the situation were simply wearing away at my loved ones.

On Tuesday, Holley had called Dr. Jay Loeffler, my former partner in developing the stereotactic radiosurgery program at the Brigham & Women's Hospital in Boston. Jay was then the chairman of radiation oncology at Massachusetts General Hospital, and Holley figured he'd be in as good a position as anyone to give her some answers.

As Holley described my situation, Jay assumed she must have been getting the details of my case wrong. What she was describing to him was, he knew, essentially impossible. But once Holley finally had him convinced that I really was in a coma caused by a rare case of *E. coli* bacterial meningitis that no one could explain the origins of, he got started calling infectious disease experts around the country. No one he spoke to had heard of a case like mine. Going over the medical literature back to 1991, he couldn't find a single case of *E. coli* meningitis in an adult who hadn't recently been through a neurosurgical procedure.

From Tuesday on, Jay called at least once a day to get an update from Phyllis or Holley and give them feedback on what his investigations had revealed. Steve Tatter, another good friend and neurosurgeon, likewise provided daily calls offering advice and comfort. But day after day, the only revelation was that my situation was the first of its kind in medical history. Spontaneous *E. coli* bacterial meningitis is rare in adults. Less than 1 in 10 million of the world's population contracts it annually.

And, like all varieties of gram-negative bacterial meningitis, it's highly aggressive. So aggressive that of the people it does attack, more than 90 percent of those who initially suffer from a rapid neurologic decline, as I did, die. And that was the mortality rate when I first entered the ER. That dismal 90 percent crept toward 100 percent as the week wore on and my body failed to respond to the antibiotics. The few who survive a case as severe as mine generally require round-the-clock care for the rest of their lives. Officially, my status was "N of 1," a term that refers to medical studies in which a single patient stands for the entire trial. There is simply no one else to whom the doctors could compare my case.

Beginning on Wednesday, Holley brought Bond in for a visit every afternoon after school. But by Friday she was starting to wonder if these visits were doing more harm than good. At times, early in the week, I would move. My body would thrash around wildly. A nurse would rub my head and give me more sedation, and eventually I'd become quiet again. This was confusing and painful for my ten-year-old son to watch. It was bad enough that he was looking at a body that no longer resembled his father, but also seeing that body make mechanical movements that he didn't recognize as mine was particularly challenging. Day by day, I became less the person he'd known, and more an unrecognizable body in a bed: a cruel and alien twin of the father he once knew.

By the end of the week these occasional bursts of motor activity had all but ceased. I needed no more sedation, because movement—even the dead, automatic kind initiated by the most primitive reflex loops of my lower brainstem and spinal cord—had dwindled almost to nil.

More family members and friends were calling, asking if

they should come. By Thursday, it had been decided that they shouldn't. There was already too much commotion in my ICU room. The nurses suggested strongly that my brain needed rest—the quieter, the better.

There was also a noticeable change in the tone of these phone calls. They too were shifting subtly from the hopeful to the hopeless. At times, looking around, Holley felt like she had lost me already.

On Thursday afternoon, Michael Sullivan got a knock on his door. It was his secretary at St. John's Episcopal Church.

"The hospital is on the line," she said. "One of the nurses taking care of Eben needs to speak with you. She says it's urgent."

Michael picked up the phone.

"Michael," the nurse told him, "you need to come right away. Eben is dying."

As a pastor, Michael had been in this situation before. Pastors see death and the wreckage it leaves behind almost as often as doctors do. Still, Michael was shocked to hear the actual word "dying" said in reference to me. He called his wife, Page, and asked her to pray: both for me, and for the strength on his part to rise to the occasion. Then he drove through the cold steady rain to the hospital, struggling to see through the tears filling his eyes.

When he got to my room the scene was much the same as it had been the last time he had visited. Phyllis was sitting by my side, taking her shift in the vigil of holding my hand that had been going on without a break since her arrival on Monday night. My chest rose and fell twelve times a minute with the ventilator, and the ICU nurse went quietly about her routine, orbiting among the machines that surrounded my bed and noting their readouts.

Another nurse came in, and Michael asked if she'd been the one who called his assistant.

"No," she replied. "I've been here all morning, and his condition has not changed much from last night. I don't know who called you."

By eleven, Holley, Mom, Phyllis, and Betsy were all in my room. Michael suggested a prayer. Everyone, including the two nurses, joined hands around the bed, and Michael made one more heartfelt plea for my return to health.

"Lord, bring Eben back to us. I know it's in your power."

Still, no one knew who had called Michael. But whoever it was, it's a good thing they did. Because the prayers coming to me from the world below—the world I'd started out from—were finally starting to get through.

18.

To Forget, and to Remember

My awareness was larger now. So large, it seemed to take in the entire universe. Have you ever listened to a song on a static-filled radio station? You get used to it. Then someone adjusts the dial and you hear the same song in its full clarity. How could you have failed to notice how dim, how far away, how entirely untrue to the original it was before?

Of course, that's how the mind works. Humans are built to adapt. I'd explained to my patients many times that this or that discomfort would lessen, or at least seem to lessen, as their bodies and brains adapted to the new situation. Something goes on long enough, and your brain learns to ignore it, or work around it, or just to treat it as normal.

But our limited earthly consciousness is far from simply normal, and I was getting my first illustration of this as I traveled ever deeper, to the very heart of the Core. I still remembered nothing of my earthly past, and yet I was not the less for this. Even though I'd forgotten my life down here, I had remembered who I really and truly was out there. I was a citizen of a universe staggering in its vastness and complexity, and ruled entirely by love.

In an almost eerie way, my discoveries beyond the body echoed the lessons I had learned just a year earlier through reconnecting with my birth family. Ultimately, none of us are orphans. We are all in the position I was, in that we have *other family:* beings who are watching and looking out for us—beings we have momentarily forgotten, but who, if we open ourselves to their presence, are waiting to help us navigate our time here on earth. None of us are ever unloved. Each and every one of us is deeply known and cared for by a Creator who cherishes us beyond any ability we have to comprehend. That knowledge must no longer remain a secret.

19

Nowhere to Hide

By Friday, my body had been on triple intravenous antibiotics for four full days but still wasn't responding. Family and friends had come from all over, and those who hadn't come had initiated prayer groups at their churches. My sister-in-law Peggy and Holley's close friend Sylvia arrived that afternoon. Holley greeted them with as cheerful a face as she could muster. Betsy and Phyllis continued to champion the *he's-going-to-be-fine* view: to remain positive at all costs. But each day it got harder to believe. Even Betsy herself began to wonder if her *no negativity in the room* order really meant something more like *no reality in the room.*

"Do you think Eben would do this for us, if the roles were reversed?" Phyllis asked Betsy that morning, after another largely sleepless night.

"What do you mean?" asked Betsy.

"I mean do you think he'd be spending every minute with us, camping out in the ICU?"

Betsy had the most beautiful, simple answer, delivered as a question: "Is there anywhere else in the world where you can imagine being?"

Both agreed that though I'd have been there in a second if needed, it was very, very hard to imagine me just sitting in one place for hours on end. "It never felt like a chore or something that had to be done—it was where we belonged," Phyllis told me later.

What was upsetting Sylvia the most were my hands and feet, which were beginning to curl up, like leaves on a plant without water. This is normal with victims of stroke and coma, as the dominant muscles in the extremities start to contract. But it's never easy for family and loved ones to see. Looking at me, Sylvia kept telling herself to stay with her original gut feeling. But even for her, it was getting very, very hard.

Holley had taken to blaming herself more and more (if only she had walked up the stairs sooner, if only this, if only that ...) and everyone worked especially hard to keep her away from the subject.

By now, everyone knew that even if I did make a recovery, *recovery* wasn't much of a word for what it would amount to. I'd need at least three months of intensive rehabilitation, would have chronic speech problems (if I had enough brain capacity to be able to speak at all), and I'd require chronic nursing care for the rest of my life. This was the best-case scenario, and as low and grim as that sounds, it was essentially in the realm of fantasy anyhow. The odds that I'd even be in that good of a shape were shrinking to nonexistent.

Bond had been kept from hearing the full details of my condition. But on Friday, at the hospital after school, he overheard one of my doctors outlining to Holley what she already knew.

It was time to face the facts. There was little room for hope.

That evening, when it was time for him to go home, Bond refused to leave my room. The regular drill was to allow only two people in my room at a time so that the doctors and nurses could work. Around six o'clock, Holley gently suggested that it was time to go home for the evening. But Bond wouldn't get up from his chair, just beneath his drawing of the battle between the white blood cell soldiers and the invading *E. coli* troops.

"He doesn't know I'm here anyway," Bond said, in a tone half bitter and half pleading. "Why can't I just stay?"

So for the rest of the evening everyone took turns coming in one at a time so Bond could stay where he was.

But the next morning—Saturday—Bond reversed his position. For the first time that week, when Holley stuck her head into his room to rouse him, he told her he didn't want to go to the hospital.

"Why not?" Holley asked.

"Because," Bond said, "I'm scared."

It was an admission that spoke for everyone.

Holley went back down to the kitchen for a few minutes. Then she tried again, asking him if he was sure he didn't want to go see his daddy.

There was a long pause as he stared at her.

"Okay," he agreed, finally.

Saturday passed with the ongoing vigil around my bed and the hopeful conversations between family and doctors. It all seemed like a half-hearted attempt to keep hope alive. Everyone's reserves were more empty than they'd been the day before.

On Saturday night, after taking our mother, Betty, back to her hotel room, Phyllis stopped by our house. It was pitch dark, with not a light in a window, and as she slogged through the soaking mud it was hard for her to keep to the flagstones. By now it had been raining for five days straight, ever since the afternoon of my entrance into the ICU. Relentless rain like this was very unusual for the highlands of Virginia, where in November it is usually crisp, clear, and sunny, like the previous Sunday, the last day before my attack. Now that day seemed so long ago, and it felt like the sky had *always* been spewing rain. When would it ever stop?

Phyllis unlocked the door and switched on the lights. Since the beginning of the week, people had been coming by and dropping off food, and though the food was still coming in, the half-hopeful/half-worried atmosphere of rallying for a temporary emergency had turned darker and more desperate. Our friends, like our family, knew that the time of any hope for me at all was nearing its end.

For a second, Phyllis thought of lighting a fire, but right on the heels of that thought came another, unwelcome one. *Why bother?* She suddenly felt more exhausted and depressed than she could ever remember feeling. She lay down on the couch in the wood-paneled study and fell into a deep sleep.

Half an hour later, Sylvia and Peggy returned, tiptoeing by the study when they saw Phyllis collapsed there. Sylvia went down to the basement and found that someone had left the freezer door open. Water was forming a puddle on the floor, and the food was starting to thaw, including several nice steaks.

When Sylvia reported the basement flood situation to Peggy, they decided to make the most of it. They made calls to the rest of the family and a few friends and got to work. Peggy went out and picked up some more side dishes, and they whipped up an impromptu feast. Soon Betsy, her daughter Kate, and her husband, Robbie, joined them, along with Bond. There was a lot of nervous chatter, and a lot of dancing around the subject on everyone's mind: that I—the absent guest of honor—would most likely never return to this house again.

Holley had returned to the hospital to continue the endless vigil. She sat by my bed, holding my hand, and kept repeating the mantras suggested by Susan Reintjes, forcing herself to stay with the meaning of the words as she said them and to believe in her heart that they were true.

"Receive the prayers.

"You have healed others. Now is your time to be healed.

"You are loved by many.

"Your body knows what to do. It is not yet your time to die."

20

The Closing

Each time I found myself stuck again in the coarse Earthworm's-Eye View, I was able to remember the brilliant Spinning Melody, which opened the portal back to the Gateway and the Core. I spent great stretches of time—which paradoxically felt like no time at all—in the presence of my guardian angel on the butterfly's wing and an eternity learning lessons from the Creator and the Orb of light deep in the Core.

At some point, I came up to the edge of the Gateway and found that I could not reenter it. The Spinning Melody—up to then my ticket into those higher regions—would no longer take me there. The gates of Heaven were closed.

Once again, describing what this felt like is challenging in the extreme, thanks to the bottleneck of linear language that we have to force everything through here on earth, and the general flattening of experience that happens when we're in the body. Think of every time you've ever experienced disappointment. There is a sense in which all the losses that we undergo here on earth are in truth variations of one absolutely central loss: the loss of Heaven. On the day that the doors of Heaven were closed to me, I felt a sense of sadness unlike any I'd ever known. Emotions are different up there. All the human emotions are present, but they're deeper, more spacious—they're not just inside but outside as well. Imagine that every time your mood changed here on earth, the weather changed instantly along with it. That your tears would bring on a torrential downpour and your joy would make the clouds instantly disappear. That gives a hint of how much more vast and consequential changes of mood feel like up there, how strangely and powerfully what we think of as "inside" and "outside" don't really exist at all.

So it was that I, heartbroken, now sank into a world of ever-increasing sorrow, a gloom that was at the same time an *actual* sinking.

I moved down through great walls of clouds. There was murmuring all around me, but I couldn't understand the words. Then I realized that countless beings were surrounding me, kneeling in arcs that spread into the distance. Looking back on it now, I realize what these half-seen, half-sensed hierarchies of beings, stretching out into the dark above and below, were doing.

They were praying for me.

Two of the faces I remembered later were those of Michael Sullivan and his wife, Page. I recall seeing them in profile only, but I clearly identified them after my return when language came back. Michael had physically been in the ICU room leading prayers numerous times, but Page was never physically there (although she had said prayers for me too).

These prayers gave me energy. That's probably why, profoundly sad as I was, something in me felt a strange confidence that everything would be all right. These beings knew I was undergoing a transition, and they were singing and praying to help me keep my spirits up. I was headed into the unknown, but by that point I had complete faith and trust that I would be taken care of, as my companion on the butterfly wing and the infinitely loving Deity had promised—that wherever I went, Heaven would come with me. It would come in the form of the Creator, of Om, and it would come in the form of the angel—my angel—the Girl on the Butterfly Wing.

I was on the way back, but I was not alone—and I knew I'd never feel alone again.

21

The Rainbow

Thinking about it later, Phyllis said that the one thing she remembered above all else about that week was the rain. A cold, driving rain from low-hanging clouds that never let up and never let the sun peek through. But then, that Sunday morning as she pulled her car into the hospital parking lot, something strange happened. Phyllis had just read a text message from one of the prayer groups in Boston saying, "Expect a miracle." As she pondered just how much of a miracle she should expect, she helped Mom step out of their car, and they both commented that the rain had stopped. To the east, the sun was shooting its rays through a chink in the cloud cover, lighting up the lovely ancient mountains to the west and the layer of cloud above as well, giving the gray clouds a golden tinge.

Then, looking toward the distant peaks, opposite to where the mid-November sun was starting its ascent, there it was.

A perfect rainbow.

Sylvia drove to the hospital with Holley and Bond for a pre-arranged meeting with my main doctor, Scott Wade. Dr. Wade was also a friend and a neighbor and had been wrestling with the worst decision that doctors dealing with life-threatening illnesses ever face. The longer I stayed in coma, the more likely it became that I would spend the rest of my life in a "persistent vegetative state." Given the high likelihood that I might still succumb to the meningitis if they simply stopped the antibiotics, it might be more sensible to cease using them—rather than to continue treatment in the face of almost certain lifelong coma. Given that my meningitis had not responded at all well to treatment, they were running the risk that they might finally eradicate my meningitis, only to enable me to live for months or years as a once-vital, now-unresponsive body, with zero quality of life.

"Have a seat," Dr. Wade told Sylvia and Holley in a tone that was kind but also unmistakably grim.

"Dr. Brennan and I have each had conference calls with experts at Duke, the University of Virginia, and Bowman Gray medical schools, and I have to tell you that everyone to a person is in agreement that things do not look good. If Eben doesn't show some real improvement within the next twelve hours, we will probably recommend discussing termination of antibiotics. A week in coma with severe bacterial meningitis is already beyond the limits of any reasonable expectation of recovery. Given those prospects, it might be better to let nature take its course."

"But, I saw his eyelids move yesterday," Holley protested. "Really, they moved. Almost like he was trying to open them. I am sure of what I saw."

"I don't doubt you did," said Dr. Wade. "His white blood cell count has come down as well. That's all good news, and I don't for a minute want to suggest that it isn't. But you need to see the situation in context. We've lightened Eben's sedation considerably, and by this point his neurologic examination should be showing more neurological activity than it is. His lower brain is partially functioning, but it's his higher-level functions that we need, and they're all still completely absent. A certain amount of improvement in apparent alertness occurs in most coma patients over time. Their bodies do things that can make it appear that they're coming back. But they're not. It's simply the brainstem moving into a state called *coma vigile*, a kind of holding pattern that they can stay in for months, or years. That's what the fluttering eyelids are, most likely. And I have to tell you again that seven days is an enormously long time to be in coma with bacterial meningitis."

Dr. Wade was using a lot of words in an attempt to soften the blow of a piece of news that could have been spoken in a single sentence.

It was time to let my body die.

22

Six Faces

A s I descended, more faces bubbled out of the muck, just as they always did when I was moving down into the Realm of the Earthworm's-Eye View. But there was something different about the faces this time. They were human now, not animal.

And they were very clearly saying things.

Not that I could make out what they were saying. It was a bit like the old Charlie Brown cartoons, when the adults speak and all you hear are indecipherable sounds. Later, upon looking back on it, I realized I could actually identify six of the faces that I saw. There was Sylvia, there was Holley, and her sister Peggy. There was Scott Wade, and there was Susan Reintjes. Of these, the only one who was not actually physically present at my bedside in those final hours was Susan. But in her way, she had, of course, been by my bedside, too, because that night, as the night before, she had sat down in her home in Chapel Hill and willed herself into my presence.

Later, learning about this, I was puzzled that my mother Betty and my sisters, who had been there all week, holding my hand lovingly for endless hours, were absent from this array of faces I'd seen. Mom had been suffering from a stress fracture in her foot, using a walker to ambulate, but she had faithfully taken her turn in the vigil. Phyllis, Betsy, and Jean had all been there. Then I learned that they had not been present that final night. The faces I remembered were those who were physically there the seventh morning of my coma, or the evening before.

Again, though, at the time, as I made the descent, I had no names or identities to attach to any of these faces. I only knew, or sensed, that they were important to me in some way.

One more in particular drew me toward it with special power. It began to tug at me. With a jolt that seemed to echo up and down the whole vast well of clouds and praying angelic beings through which I was descending, I suddenly realized that the beings of the Gateway and the Core—beings I had known and loved, seemingly, forever—were not the only beings I knew. I knew, and loved, beings down below me, too—down in the realm I was fast approaching. Beings I had, until now, completely forgotten.

This knowledge focused on all six faces, but in particular on the sixth one. It was so familiar. I realized with a feeling of shock bordering on absolute fear that whoever it was, it was the face of someone who needed me. Someone who would never recover if I left. If I abandoned it, the loss would be unbearable—like the feeling I'd gotten when the gates to Heaven had closed. It would be a betrayal I simply couldn't commit.

Up to that point, I had been free. I had journeyed through worlds in the way that adventurers most effectively can: without any real concern about their fate. The outcome didn't ultimately matter, because even when I was in the Core, there was never any worry or guilt about letting anyone down. That had, of course, been one of the first things that I'd learned when I was with the Girl on the Butterfly Wing and she'd told me: "There is nothing you can do that is wrong."

But now it was different. So different that, for the first time in my entire voyage, I felt remarkable terror. It was a terror not for myself, but for these faces—in particular for that sixth face. A face that I still couldn't identify, but that I knew was crucially important to me.

This face took on ever greater detail, until at last I saw that it—that *he*—was actually pleading for me to return: to risk the terrible descent into the world below to be with him again. I still could not understand his words, but somehow they conveyed that I had a stake in this world below—that I had, as they say, "skin in the game."

It mattered that I returned. I had ties here—ties that I had to honor. The clearer the face became, the more I realized this. And the closer I came to recognizing the face.

The face of a young boy.

23

Final Night, First Morning

Before sitting down with Dr. Wade, Holley told Bond to wait outside the door because she hadn't wanted him to hear what she feared was very bad news. But sensing this, Bond had lingered outside the door and caught some of Dr. Wade's words. Enough of them to understand the real situation. To understand that his father was not, in fact, coming back. Ever.

Bond ran into the room and up to my bed. Sobbing, he kissed my forehead and rubbed my shoulders. Then he pulled up my eyelids and said, directly into my empty, unfocused eyes, "You're going to be okay, Daddy. You're going to be okay." He kept on repeating it, again and again, believing, in his child's way, that if he said it enough times, surely he would make it true.

Meanwhile, in a room down the hall, Holley stared into space, absorbing Dr. Wade's words as best she could.

Finally, she said, "I guess that means I should call Eben at college and have him come back."

Dr. Wade didn't deliberate on the question.

"Yes, I think that would be the right thing to do."

Holley walked over to the conference room's large picture window, which looked out on the storm-soaked but brightening Virginia mountains, took out her cell phone, and dialed Eben's number.

As she did so, Sylvia stood up from her chair.

"Holley, wait a minute," she said. "Let me just go in there one more time."

Sylvia went into the ICU room and stood by the bed next to Bond, as he sat silently rubbing my hand. Sylvia put her hand on my arm and stroked it gently. As it had been all week, my head was turned slightly to one side. For a week, everyone had been looking *at* my face, rather than into it. The only time my eyes opened was when the doctors checked for pupil dilation in reaction to light (one of the simplest but most effective ways to check for brainstem function), or when Holley or Bond, against the doctors' repeated instructions, had insisted on doing so and encountered two eyes staring dead and unmoored, askew like those of a broken doll.

But now, as Sylvia and Bond stared into my slack face, resolutely refusing to accept what they had just heard from the doctor, something happened.

My eyes opened.

Sylvia shrieked. She would later tell me that the next biggest shock, almost as shocking as my eyes opening, was the way they immediately began to look around. Up, down, here, there . . . They reminded her not of an adult emerging from a seven-day coma, but of an infant—someone newly born to the world, looking around at it, taking it in for the first time.

In a way, she was right.

Sylvia recovered from her initial flat-out shock and realized that I was agitated by something. She ran out of the room to where Holley was still standing at the big picture window, talking to Eben IV.

"Holley . . . Holley!" Sylvia shouted. "He's awake. Awake! Tell Eben his dad is coming back."

Holley stared at Sylvia. "Eben," she said into the phone, "I have to call you back. He's . . . your father is coming back . . . to life."

Holley walked, then ran into the ICU, with Dr. Wade right

behind her. Sure enough, I was thrashing around on the bed. Not mechanically, but because I was conscious, and something was clearly bothering me. Dr. Wade immediately understood what it was: the breathing tube that was still in my throat. The tube I no longer needed, because my brain, along with the rest of my body, had just kicked back to life. He reached over, cut the securing tape, and carefully extracted it.

I choked a little, gasped down my first fully unaided lungful of air in seven days, and spoke the first words I'd spoken in a week as well:

"Thank you."

Phyllis was still thinking about the rainbow she'd just seen when she exited the elevator. She was pushing Mom in a wheelchair. They walked into the room, and Phyllis almost fell over backward in disbelief. I was sitting up in my bed, meeting their gaze with my own. Betsy was jumping up and down. She hugged Phyllis. They were both in tears. Phyllis came closer and looked deep into my eyes.

I looked back at her, then around at everyone else.

As my loving family and caregivers gathered around my bed, still dumbstruck by the inexplicable transition, I had a peaceful, joyous smile.

"All is well," I said, radiating that blissful message as much as speaking the words. I looked at each of them, deeply, acknowledging the divine miracle of our very existence.

"Don't worry . . . all is well," I repeated, to assuage any doubt. Phyllis told me later that it was as if I were imparting a crucial message from the beyond, that the world is as it should be, that we have nothing to fear. She said she often recalls that moment when she is vexed by some earthly concern—to find comfort in knowing that we are never alone.

As I took stock of the entourage, I seemed to be returning to my earthly existence.

"What," I asked those who were assembled, "are you doing here?"

To which Phyllis replied, "What are *you* doing here?"

24

The Return

Bond had envisioned his same old dad would wake up, take a look around, and just need a little catching up on what had happened before resuming my role as the father he'd always known.

He soon discovered, however, that it wasn't going to be quite that easy. Dr. Wade cautioned Bond about two things: First, he shouldn't count on my remembering anything I was saying as I emerged from the coma. He explained that the process of memory takes enormous brain power, and that my brain wasn't sufficiently recovered to be performing at that sophisticated level. Second, he shouldn't worry much about what I said during these early days, because a lot of it was going to sound pretty crazy.

He proved right on both counts.

That first morning back, Bond proudly showed me the drawing he and Eben IV had made of my white blood cells attacking the *E. coli* bacteria.

"Wow, wonderful," I said.

Bond glowed with pride and excitement.

Then I continued: "What are the conditions like outside? What does the computer readout say? You need to move, I'm getting ready to jump!"

Bond's face fell. Needless to say, this was not the full return he had been hoping for.

I was having wild delusions, reliving some of the most exciting times of my life, in the most vivid fashion.

In my mind, I was on jump run, ready to skydive out of a DC3 three miles above the earth . . . going to be the last man out, my favorite position. It was the maximal flying of my body.

Bursting into brilliant sunshine outside the airplane door, I immediately assumed a head dive with my arms tucked behind me (in my mind), feeling the familiar buffeting as I fell beneath the prop blast, watching from upside down as the belly of the enormous silvery plane started to shoot skyward, its huge propellers whirling in slow motion, earth and clouds below mirrored on its underbelly. I was musing over the odd sight of flaps and wheels down (as if landing) while still miles above the ground (all to slow down and minimize wind shock to the exiting jumpers).

I tucked my arms in extra tight in a head-down dive to accelerate briskly to over 220 miles per hour, nothing more than my speckled blue helmet and shoulders against thin upper air to resist the tug of the huge planet below, moving more than the length of a football field every second, the wind roaring by furiously at thrice hurricane speed, louder than anything—ever.

Passing between the tops of two enormous puffy white clouds, I rocketed into the clear chasm between them, green earth and sparkling deep blue sea far below, in my wild, thrilling rush down to join my friends, just barely visible, in the colorful snowflake formation, growing larger every second as other jumpers joined in, far, far below . . .

I was flipping back and forth between being present there in the ICU and being out of my mind in the adrenaline-soaked delusions of a gorgeous skydive.

I was between nutty—and getting it.

For two days I blabbered about skydiving, airplanes, and the Internet to all who would listen. As my physical brain gradually recovered its bearings, I entered a strange and exhausting paranoid universe. I became obsessed with an ugly background of "Internet messages" that would show up whenever I closed my eyes, and that sometimes appeared on the ceiling when they were open. When I shut my eyes I heard grinding, monotonous, anti-melodious chanting sounds that usually went away when I opened them again. I kept putting my finger in the air, pointing just like ET, trying to guide the Internet ticker flowing past me, in Russian, Chinese.

In short, I was a little crazy.

It was all a little like the Realm of the Earthworm's-Eye View, only more nightmarish, because what I heard and saw was laced with the trappings of my human past (I recognized my family members, even when, as in Holley's case, I didn't remember their names).

But at the same time it completely lacked the astonishing clarity and vibrant richness—the ultra-reality—of the Gateway and the Core. I was most definitely back in my brain.

Despite that initial moment of seemingly full lucidity when my eyes first opened, I soon once again had no memory of my human life before coma. My only memory was of where I had just been: the rough, ugly Realm of the Earthworm's-Eye View, the idyllic Gateway, and the awesome heavenly Core. My mind—my real self—was squeezing its way back into the all too tight and limiting suit of physical existence, with its spatio-temporal bounds, its linear thought, and its limitation to verbal communication. Things that up until a week ago I'd thought were the only mode of existence around, but which now showed themselves as extraordinarily cumbersome limitations.

Physical life is characterized by defensiveness, whereas spiritual life is just the opposite. This is the only explanation I could come up with to explain why my reentry had such a strong paranoid aspect to it. For a stretch of time I became convinced that Holley (whose name I still didn't know but whom I somehow recognized as my wife) and my physicians were trying to kill me. I had further dreams and fantasies about flight and skydiving—some of them extremely long and involved. In the longest, most intense, and almost ridiculously detailed of these, I found myself in a South Florida cancer clinic featuring outdoor escalators where I was pursued by Holley, two South Florida police officers, and a pair of Asian ninja photographers on cable pulleys.

I was in fact going through something called "ICU psychosis." It's normal, even expected, for patients whose brains are coming back online after being inactive for a long period. I'd seen it many a time, but never from the inside. And from the inside it was very, very different indeed.

The most interesting thing about this session of nightmares and paranoid fantasies, in retrospect, is that all of it was indeed that: a fantasy. Portions of it—in particular the extended South Florida ninja nightmare—were extremely intense, and even outright terrifying while happening. But in retrospect—indeed, almost immediately after this period ended—it all became clearly recognizable as what it was: something cooked up by my very beleaguered brain as it was trying to recover its bearings. Some of the dreams I had during this period were stunningly and frighteningly vivid. But in the end they served only to underline how very, very dissimilar my dream state had been compared with the ultra-reality deep in coma.

As for the rockets, airplanes, and skydiving themes that I imagined so consistently, they were, I later realized, quite accurate from a symbolic point of view. Because the fact was that

I *was* making a dangerous reentry from a place far away, to the abandoned but now once again functional space station of my brain. One could hardly ask for a better earthly analogy for what happened to me during my week out of body than a rocket launch.

25

Not There Yet

B ond wasn't the only one having difficulty accepting the decidedly kooky person I was during those first days back. The day after I recovered consciousness—Monday—Phyllis called Eben IV on his computer using Skype.

"Eben, here's your dad," she said, turning the video camera toward me.

"Hi, Dad! How's it going?" he said cheerfully.

For a minute I just grinned and stared at the computer screen. When I finally spoke, Eben was crushed. I was painfully slow in my speech, and the words themselves made little sense. Eben later told me, "You sounded like a zombie—like someone on a bad acid trip." Unfortunately, he had not been forewarned about the possibility of an ICU psychosis.

Gradually my paranoia abated, and my thinking and conversation became more lucid. Two days after my awakening, I was transferred to the Neuroscience Step-down Unit. The nurses there gave Phyllis and Betsy cots so that they could sleep next to me. I trusted no one but the two of them—they made me feel safe, tethered to my new reality.

The only problem was that I didn't sleep. I kept them up all night, going on about the Internet, space stations, Russian double agents, and all manner of related nonsense. Phyllis tried to convince the nurses that I had a cough, hoping a little cough syrup would bring on an hour or so of uninterrupted sleep. I was like a newborn who did not adhere to a sleep schedule.

In my quieter moments, Phyllis and Betsy helped pull me slowly back to earth. They recalled all kinds of stories from our childhood, and though by and large I listened as if I were hearing them for the first time, I was fascinated all the same. The more they talked, the more something important began to glimmer inside me—the realization that I had, in fact, been there for these events myself.

Very quickly, both sisters told me later, the brother they had known became visible again, through the thick fog of paranoid chatter.

"It was amazing," Betsy later told me. "You were just coming out of coma, you weren't at all fully aware of where you were or what was going on, you talked about all kinds of crazy stuff half the time, and yet your sense of humor was just fine. It was obviously *you*. You were back!"

"One of the first things you did was crack a joke about feeding yourself," Phyllis later confided. "We were prepared to have fed you spoonful by spoonful for as long as it took. But you'd have none of it. You were determined to get that orange Jell-O into your mouth on your own."

As the temporarily stunned engines of my brain kicked back in ever further, I would watch myself say or do things and marvel: where did *that* come from? Early on, a Lynchburg friend named Jackie came by to visit. Holley and I had known Jackie and her husband, Ron, well, having bought our house from them. Without my willing them to do so, my deeply ingrained southern social graces kicked in. Seeing Jackie, I immediately asked, "How's Ron?"

After a few more days, I started having occasional genuinely lucid conversations with my visitors, and again it was fascinating to see how much of these connections were automatic and did not require much effort on my part. Like a jet on autopilot, my brain somehow negotiated these increasingly familiar landscapes of human experience. I was getting a firsthand demonstration of a truth that I'd known very well as a neurosurgeon: the brain is a truly marvelous mechanism.

Of course, the unspoken question on everybody's mind (including mine in my more lucid moments) was: How well would I get? Was I really returning in full, or had the *E. coli* done at least some of the damage all the doctors had been sure it would do? This daily waiting tore at everyone, especially Holley, who feared that all of a sudden the miraculous progress would stop, and she would be left with only a portion of the "me" she had known.

Yet day by day, ever more of that "me" returned. Language. Memories. Recognition. A certain mischievous streak I've always been known for returned as well. And while they were pleased to see my sense of humor back, my two sisters weren't always thrilled with how I chose to use it. Monday afternoon, Phyllis touched my forehead and I recoiled.

"Ouch," I screamed. "That hurts!"

Then, after enjoying everybody's horrified expressions, I said, "Just kidding."

Everyone was surprised by the speed of my recovery—except for me. I—as of yet—had no real clue how close to death I had actually been. As, one by one, friends and family headed back to their lives, I wished them well and remained blissfully ignorant of the tragedy that had been so narrowly averted. I was so ebullient that one of the neurologists who evaluated me for rehab placement insisted that I was "too euphoric," and that I was probably suffering from brain damage. This doctor, like me, was a regular bow-tie wearer, and I returned the favor of his diagnosis by telling my sisters, after he had left, that he was "strangely flat of affect for a bow-tie aficionado."

Even then, I knew something that more and more of the people around me would come to accept as well. Doctors' views or no doctors' views, I wasn't sick, or brain-damaged. I was completely well.

In fact—though at this point only I knew this—I was completely and truly "well" for the first time in my entire life.

26

Spreading the News

"Truly well"—even if I did still have some work to do as far as the hardware side of things went. A few days after moving to outpatient rehab, I called Eben IV at school. He mentioned that he was working on a paper in one of his neuroscience courses. I volunteered to help but soon regretted doing so. It was much harder for me to focus on the subject than I had expected, and terminology I thought I had fully back suddenly refused to come to my mind. I realized with a shock just how far I still had to go.

But bit by bit that part came back, too. I'd wake up one day and find myself in possession of whole continents of scientific and medical knowledge that the day before I had been without. It was one of the strangest aspects of my experience: opening my eyes in the morning with even more of the nuts and bolts of a whole lifetime of education and experience at work again.

While my neuroscientist's knowledge crept back slowly and timidly, my memories of what had happened during that week out of my body loomed in my memory with astonishing boldness and clarity. What had happened outside the earthly realm had everything to do with the wild happiness I'd awakened with, and the bliss that continued to stick with me. I was deliriously happy because I was back with the people I loved. But I was also happy because—to state the matter as plainly as I can—I understood for the first time who I really was, and what kind of a world we inhabit.

I was wildly—and naïvely—eager to share these experiences, especially with my fellow doctors. After all, what I'd undergone altered my long-held beliefs of what the brain is, what consciousness is, even what life itself means—and doesn't mean. Who wouldn't be anxious to hear of my discoveries?

Quite a few people, as it turned out. Most especially, people with medical degrees.

Make no mistake, my doctors were very happy for me. "That's wonderful, Eben," they would say, echoing my response to countless patients of my own who, in the past, had tried to tell me about otherworldly experiences they'd undergone during surgery. "You were very sick. Your brain was soaking in pus. We can't believe you're even here to talk about it. You know yourself what the brain can come up with when it's that far gone."

In short, they couldn't wrap their minds around what I was so desperately trying to share.

But then, how could I blame them? After all, I certainly wouldn't have understood it either—*before*.

27

Homecoming

I came home on November 25, 2008, two days before Thanks-giving, to a home full of gratitude. Eben IV drove overnight to surprise me the following morning. The last time he'd been with me I'd been in full coma, and he was still processing the fact that I was alive at all. He was so excited that he got a speeding ticket coming through Nelson County just north of Lynchburg.

I'd been up for hours, sitting in my easy chair by the fire in our cozy wood-paneled study, just thinking about everything I'd been through. Eben walked through the door just after 6 A.M. I stood up and gave him a long hug. He was stunned. The last time he'd seen me on Skype in the hospital, I'd been barely able to form a sentence. Now—other than still being on the thin side and having an IV line in my arm—I had returned to my favorite role in life—being Eben and Bond's dad.

Well, almost the same. Eben *was* aware of something else that was different about me, too. Later, Eben would say that when he first saw me that day, he was immediately taken with how "present" I was.

"You were so clear, so focused," he said. "It was as if there was a kind of light shining within you."

I wasted no time in sharing my thoughts.

"I am so eager to read all I can about this," I told him. "It was all so real, Eben, almost *too* real to be real, if that makes any sense. I want to write about it for other neuroscientists.

And I want to read up on NDEs and what other people have experienced. I can't believe I never took any of it seriously, never listened to what my own patients told me. I was never curious enough to even look into any of the literature."

Eben didn't say anything, at first, but it was clear he was thinking about how to best advise his dad. He sat down across from me, and he urged me to see what should have been obvious.

"I believe you, Dad," he said. "But think about it. If you want this to be of value to others, the last thing you should do is read what other people have said."

"So what should I do?" I asked.

"Write it down. Write it all down—all your memories, as accurately as you can remember them. But don't read any books or articles about other peoples' near-death experiences, or physics, or cosmology. Not until you've written down what happened to you. Don't talk to Mom or anyone else about what happened while you were in coma, either—at least to the degree that you can steer clear of it. You can do that all you want later, right? Think how you always used to tell me that observation comes first, *then* interpretation. If you want what happened to you to be scientifically valuable, you need to record it as purely and accurately as you can *before* you start making any comparisons with what has happened to others."

It was, perhaps, the most sage advice anyone's ever given me—and I followed it. Eben was also quite right that what I deeply wanted, more than anything else, was to use my experiences to, hopefully, help others. The more my scientific mind returned, the more clearly I saw how radically what I'd learned in decades of schooling and medical practice conflicted with what I'd experienced, the more I understood that the mind and the personality (as some would call it, our soul or spirit) continue to exist beyond the body. I had to tell my story to the world.

For the next six weeks or so, most days went the same. I'd wake up around 2 or 2:30 A.M., feeling so ecstatic and energized by simply being alive that I would bound out of bed. I'd light a fire in the den, sit down in my old leather chair, and write. I tried to recall every detail of my journeys in and out of the Core, and what I had felt as I learned its many life-changing lessons.

Though *tried* isn't really the right word. Crisp and clear, the memories were right there, right where I had left them.

28.

The Ultra-Real

*There are two ways to be fooled. One is to believe what isn't
true; the other is to refuse to believe what is true.*

—Søren Kierkegaard (1813–1855)

In all this writing, one word seemed to come up again and
again.

Real.

Never, before my coma, had I realized just how deceptive a
word can be. The way I had been taught to think about it, both
in medical school and in that school of common sense called
life, is that something is either real (a car accident, a football
game, a sandwich on the table in front of you) or it's not. In
my years as a neurosurgeon, I'd seen plenty of people undergo
hallucinations. I thought I knew just how terrifying unreal
phenomena could be to those experiencing them. And during
my few days of ICU psychosis, I'd had a chance to sample some
impressively realistic nightmares as well. But once they passed,
I quickly recognized those nightmares for the delusions they
were: neuronal phantasmagoria stirred up by brain circuitry
struggling to get running again.

But while I was in coma my brain hadn't been working improperly. *It hadn't been working at all.* The part of my brain that
years of medical school had taught me was responsible for creat-

ing the world I lived and moved in and for taking the raw data that came in through my senses and fashioning it into a meaningful universe: that part of my brain was down, and out. And yet despite all of this, I had been alive, and aware, *truly aware*, in a universe characterized above all by love, consciousness, and reality. (There was that word again.) There was, for me, simply no arguing this fact. I knew it so completely that I ached.

What I'd experienced was more real than the house I sat in, more real than the logs burning in the fireplace. Yet there was no room for that reality in the medically trained scientific worldview that I'd spent years acquiring.

How was I going to create room for both of these realities to coexist?

29

A Common Experience

Finally the day came when I had written down everything I could, every last memory of the Realm of the Earthworm's-Eye View, the Gateway, and the Core.

Then it was time to read. I plunged into the ocean of NDE literature—an ocean into which I'd never so much as dipped a toe before. It didn't take me long to realize that countless other people had experienced the things I had, both in recent years and centuries past. NDEs are not all the same, each one is unique—but the same elements show up again and again, and many I recognized from my own experience. Narratives of passing through a dark tunnel or valley into a bright and vivid landscape—ultra-real—were as old as ancient Greece and Egypt. Angelic beings—sometimes winged, sometimes not—went back, at least, to the ancient Near East—as did the belief that such beings were guardians who watched the activities of people on earth and greeted those people when they left it behind. The sense of being able to see in all directions simultaneously; the sensation of being above linear time—of being above *everything*, essentially, that I had previously thought of as defining the landscape of human life; the hearing of anthem-like music, which entered through one's whole being rather than simply one's ears; the direct and instantaneous reception of concepts that normally would have taken a very long time and a great deal of study to comprehend, without any struggle whatsoever . . . feeling the intensity of unconditional love.

Over and over, in the modern NDE accounts and in spiritual writings from earlier times, I'd feel the narrator struggling with the limitations of earthly language, trying to get the entirety of the fish they had hooked on board the boat of human language and ideas . . . and always, to one degree or another, failing.

And yet, with each attempt that fell frustratingly short of its goal, each person straining at language and ideas to get this enormity across to the reader, I'd understand the aim of the storyteller and what they'd hoped to convey in all of its boundaryless majesty, but simply couldn't.

Yes, yes, yes! I'd say to myself as I read. *I understand.*

These books, this material, had all, of course, been there before my experience. But I'd never *looked* at it. Not just in terms of reading, but in another way as well. Quite simply, I'd never held myself open to the idea that there might be anything genuine to the idea that something of us survives the death of the body. I was the quintessential good-natured, albeit skeptical, doctor. And as such, I can tell you that most skeptics aren't really skeptics at all. To be truly skeptical, one must actually examine something, and take it seriously. And I, like many doctors, had never taken the time to explore NDEs. I had simply "known" they were impossible.

I also went through the medical records of my time in coma—a time that was meticulously recorded, practically from the very start. Reviewing my scans just as I would have for a patient of my own, it became clear to me at last just how fantastically sick I had been.

Bacterial meningitis is unique among diseases in the manner in which it attacks the outer surface of the brain while leaving its deeper structures intact. The bacteria efficiently wreck the human part of our brain first, and finally prove fatal by attacking the deeper "housekeeping" structures common to other animals, deep beneath the human part. The other conditions that can damage the neocortex and cause unconsciousness—head trauma, stroke, brain hemorrhages or brain tumors—are not nearly as efficient at completely damaging the entire surface of the neocortex. These tend to involve only part of the neocortex, leaving other parts unscathed and able to function. Not only that, but instead of taking the neocortex alone out, they tend to also damage the deeper and more primitive parts of the brain as well. Given all of this, bacterial meningitis is arguably the best disease one could find if one were seeking to mimic human death without actually bringing it about. (Though of course, it usually does. The sad truth is that virtually everyone as sick as I was from bacterial meningitis never returns to tell the tale.) (See Appendix A.)

Though the experience is as old as history, "the near-death experience" (regardless of whether it was seen as something real or a baseless fantasy) only became a household term fairly recently. In the 1960s, new techniques were developed that allowed doctors to resuscitate patients who had suffered a cardiac arrest. Patients who in former times simply would have died were now pulled back into the land of the living. Unbeknownst to them, these physicians were, through their rescue efforts, producing a breed of trans-earthly voyagers: people who had glimpsed beyond the veil and returned to tell about it. Today they number in the millions. Then, in 1975, a medical student named Raymond Moody published a book called *Life After Life*, in which he described the experience of a man named George Ritchie. Ritchie had "died" as a result of cardiac arrest as a complication of pneumonia and been out of his body for nine minutes. He traveled down a tunnel, visited heavenly and hellish regions, met a being of light that he identified as Jesus, and experienced feelings of peace and well-being that were so intense he had difficulty putting them into words. The era of the modern near-death experience was born.

I couldn't claim complete ignorance of Moody's book, but I had certainly never read it. I didn't need to, because I knew, first of all, that the idea that cardiac arrest represented some kind of close-to-death condition was nonsense. Much of the literature about near-death experiences concerns patients whose hearts stopped for a few minutes—usually after an accident or on the operating table. The idea that cardiac arrest constitutes death is outdated by about fifty years. Many laypeople still believe that if someone comes back from cardiac arrest, then they have "died" and returned to life, but the medical community long ago revised its definitions of death to center on the brain, not the heart (ever since brain death criteria, which rely on crucial findings of the patient's neurological examination, were established in 1968). Cardiac arrest is relevant to death only in terms of its effect on the brain. Within seconds of cardiac arrest, cessation of blood flow to the brain leads to widespread disruption of cooperative neural activity and loss of consciousness.

For half a century, surgeons have routinely stopped the heart for minutes to hours in cardiac surgery and occasionally neurosurgery, using cardiopulmonary bypass pumps, and sometimes cooling the brain to enhance its viability under such stresses. No brain death occurs. Even a person whose heart stops on the street might be spared brain damage, provided that someone starts performing cardiopulmonary resuscitation within four minutes and the heart can eventually be restarted. As long as oxygenated blood travels to the brain, the brain—and therefore the person—will stay alive, albeit transiently unconscious.

This piece of knowledge was all I needed to discount Moody's book without ever opening it. But now I did open it, and reading the stories Moody reported with the reference of what I myself had gone through made me completely shift my perspective. I had little doubt that at least some of the people in these stories had genuinely left their physical bodies. The similarities with what I myself had experienced beyond the body were simply too overwhelming.

The more primitive parts of my brain—the housekeeping parts—functioned for all or most of my time in coma. But when it came to the part of my brain that every single brain scientist will tell you is responsible for the human side of me: well, that part was gone. I could see it on the scans, in the lab numbers, on my neurological exams—in all the data from my very closely recorded week in hospital. I quickly began to realize that mine was a technically near-impeccable near-death experience, perhaps one of the most convincing such cases in modern history. What really mattered about my case was not what happened to me personally, but the sheer, flat-out impossibility of arguing, from a medical standpoint, that it was all fantasy.

Describing what an NDE is is challenging, at best, but doing so in the face of a medical profession that refuses to believe it's possible at all makes it even harder. Due to my career in neuroscience and my own NDE, I now had the unique opportunity to make it more palatable.

30

Back from the Dead

And the drawing near of Death, which alike levels all, alike impresses all with a last revelation, which only an author from the dead could adequately tell.

—HERMAN MELVILLE (1819–1891)

Everywhere I went in those first few weeks, people looked at me like I had risen from the grave. I ran into one doctor who had been present at the hospital the day I'd come in. He hadn't been directly involved in my care, but he'd gotten a good eyeful when I was rolled into the ER that first morning.

"How can you even *be* here?" he asked, summarizing the medical community's basic question about me. "Are you Eben's twin brother, or what?"

I smiled, reached out, and shook his hand firmly, to let him know it was really I.

Though he was of course joking about whether I had a twin brother, this doctor was actually making an important point. For all intents and purposes I still *was* two people, and if I was going to do what I'd told Eben IV I wanted to do—use my experience to help others—I would have to reconcile my NDE with my scientific understanding and knit those two people together.

My memory went back to a phone call I'd received one morning several years before, from the mother of a patient who'd called as I was examining a digital map of a tumor I was to re-move later that day. I'll call the woman Susanna. Susanna's late husband, whom I will call George, had been a patient of mine with a brain tumor. In spite of everything we did, he died within a year and a half of diagnosis. Now Susanna's daughter was ill with several brain metastases from breast cancer. Her prospects of survival beyond a few months were remote. It wasn't a good time to take a call—my mind was completely absorbed in the digital image in front of me, and with mapping out exactly what my strategy was going to be to go in and remove it without doing damage to the brain tissue around it. But I stayed on the line with Susanna because I knew that she was trying to think of something—anything—to allow her to cope.

I'd always believed that when you're under the burden of a potentially fatal illness, softening the truth is fine. To prevent a terminal patient from trying to grab on to a little fantasy to help them deal with the possibility of death is like withholding pain-killing medication. It was an extraordinarily heavy load to carry, and I owed Susanna every second of attention she asked.

"Dr. A," Susanna said, "my daughter had the most incredible dream. Her father came to her in it. He told her everything was going to be all right, that she didn't need to worry about dying."

It was the kind of thing I'd heard from patients countless times—the mind doing what it can to soothe itself in an un-bearably painful situation. I told her it sounded like a wonderful dream.

"But the most incredible thing, Dr. A, is what he was wear-ing. A yellow shirt—and a fedora!"

"Well, Susanna," I said good-naturedly, "I guess there are no dress codes in Heaven."

"No," Susanna said. "That's not it. Early on in our relationship, when we were first dating, I gave George a yellow shirt. He liked to wear it with a fedora that I also gave him. But the shirt and hat were lost when our luggage failed to arrive on our honeymoon. He already knew by that time how much I loved him in that shirt and hat, but we never replaced them."

"I'm sure Christina had heard lots of wonderful stories about that shirt and hat, Susanna," I said. "And about your early times together . . ."

"No," she laughed. "That's what's so wonderful. That was our little secret. We knew how ridiculous it would sound to someone else. We never talked about that shirt and fedora after they were lost. Christina never heard one peep from us about them. Christina was so afraid of dying, and now she knows she has nothing to fear, nothing at all.

What Susanna was telling me, I discovered in my reading, was a variety of dream confirmation that happens quite often. But I hadn't had my NDE when I'd gotten that call, and at the time I knew perfectly well that what Susanna was telling me was a grief-induced fantasy. Over the course of my career, I had treated many patients who had undergone unusual experiences while in coma or during surgery. Whenever one of these people narrated an unusual experience like Susanna's, I was always completely sympathetic. And I was quite sure these experiences had indeed happened—in their minds. The brain is the most sophisticated—and temperamental—organ we possess. Tinker around with it, lessen the degree of oxygen it gets by a few torr (a unit of pressure), and the owner of that brain is going to experience an alteration in their reality. Or, more precisely, their personal experience of reality. Throw in all the physical trauma and all the medications that someone with a brain malady is likely to be on, and you have a virtual guarantee that, should a patient have any memories when they come back around, those memories are going to be pretty unusual. With a brain affected by a deadly bacterial infection and mind-altering medications, *anything* could happen. Anything, that is—*except* the ultra-real experience I had in coma.

Susanna, I realized with the kind of jolt that comes when you see something that should have been obvious, wasn't calling to be comforted by me that day. She really and truly was trying to comfort me. But I hadn't been able to see that. I'd thought I was doing Susanna a kindness by pretending, in my wan, distracted way, to believe her story. But I wasn't. And looking back on that conversation and dozens of others like it, I realized just what a long road I had in front of me if I was going to convince my fellow doctors that what I'd been through was real.

31.

Three Camps

I maintain that the human mystery is incredibly demeaned by scientific reductionism, with its claim in promissory materialism to account eventually for all of the spiritual world in terms of patterns of neuronal activity. This belief must be classed as a superstition. . . . we have to recognize that we are spiritual beings with souls existing in a spiritual world as well as material beings with bodies and brains existing in a material world.

—Sir John C. Eccles (1903–1997)

When it came to NDEs, there were three basic camps. There were the believers: either people who had undergone an NDE themselves or who simply found such experiences easy to accept. Then, of course, there were the staunch unbelievers (like the old me). These people didn't generally classify themselves as unbelievers, however. They simply "knew" that the brain generated consciousness and wouldn't hold still for crazy ideas of mind beyond the body (unless they were good-naturedly comforting someone, as I had thought I'd been doing with Susanna that day).

Then there was the middle group. In here there were all kinds of people who had heard about NDEs, either by reading about them or—because they're extraordinarily common—by having a friend or relative who had undergone one. These people in the middle were the ones my story could really help. The news that NDEs bring is life-transforming. But when a person who is potentially open to hearing about an NDE asks a doctor or a scientist—in our society the official gatekeepers on the matter of what's real and what isn't—they are all too often told, gently but firmly, that NDEs are fantasies: products of a brain struggling to hold on to life, and nothing more.

As a doctor who'd undergone what I had, I could tell a different story. And the more I thought about it, the more I felt I had a duty to do just that.

One by one, I ran down the suggestions that I knew my colleagues, and I myself in the old days, would have offered to "explain" what happened to me. (For more details, see my summary of neuroscientific hypotheses, Appendix B.)

Was my experience a primitive brainstem program that evolved to ease terminal pain and suffering—possibly a remnant of "feigned-death" strategies used by lower mammals? I discounted that one right out of the gate. There was, quite simply, no way that my experiences, with their intensely sophisticated visual and aural levels, and their high degree of perceived meaning, were the product of the reptilian portion of my brain.

Was it a distorted recall of memories from deeper parts of my limbic system, the part of the brain that fuels emotional perception? Again, no—without a functioning neocortex the limbic system could not produce visions with the clarity and logic I experienced.

Could my experience have been a kind of psychedelic vision produced by some of the (many) drugs I was on? Again, all these drugs work with receptors in the neocortex. And with no neocortex functioning, there was no canvas for these drugs to work on.

How about REM intrusion? This is the name of a syndrome (related to "rapid eye movement" or REM sleep, the phase in which dreams occur) in which natural neurotransmitters such as serotonin interact with receptors in the neocortex. Sorry again. REM intrusion needs a functioning neocortex to happen, and I didn't have one.

Then there was the hypothetical phenomenon known as a "DMT dump." In this situation, the pineal gland, reacting to the stress of a perceived threat to the brain, produces a substance called DMT (or N,N-dimethyltryptamine). DMT is structurally similar to serotonin and can bring on an extremely intense psychedelic state. I'd had no personal experience with DMT—and still haven't—but I have no argument with those who say it can produce a very powerful psychedelic experience; maybe one with genuine implications for our understanding of what consciousness, and reality, actually are.

However, it remains a fact that the portion of the brain that DMT affects (the neocortex) was, in my case, not there to be affected. So in terms of "explaining" what happened to me, the DMT-dump hypothesis came up as radically short as the other chief candidates for explanations of my experience, and for the same key reason. Hallucinogens affect the neocortex, and my neocortex wasn't available to be affected.

The final hypothesis I looked at was that of the "reboot phenomenon." This would explain my experience as an assembly of essentially disjointed memories and thoughts left over from before my cortex went completely down. Like a computer restarting and saving what it could after a system-wide failure, my brain would have pieced together my experience from these leftover bits as best it could. This might occur on restarting the cortex into consciousness after a prolonged system-wide failure, as in my diffuse meningitis. But this seems most unlikely given the intricacies and interactivity of my elaborate recollections. Because I experienced the nonlinear nature of time in the spiritual world so intensely, I can now understand why so much writing on the spiritual dimension can seem distorted or simply nonsensical from our earthly perspective. In the worlds above this one, time simply doesn't behave as it does here. It's not necessarily one-thing-after-another in those worlds. A moment can seem like a lifetime, and one or several lifetimes can seem like a moment. But though time doesn't behave ordinarily (in our terms) in the worlds beyond, that doesn't mean it's jumbled, and my own recollections from my time in coma were anything but. My most this-worldly anchors in my experience, temporally speaking, were my interactions with Susan Reintjes when she contacted me on my fourth and fifth nights, and the appearance, toward the end of my journey, of those six faces. Any other appearance of temporal simultaneity between events on earth and my journey beyond it are, you might say, purely conjectural!

The more I learned of my condition, and the more I sought, using the current scientific literature, to explain what had happened, the more I came up spectacularly short. Everything—the uncanny clarity of my vision, the clearness of my thoughts as pure conceptual flow—suggested higher, not lower, brain functioning. But my higher brain had not been around to do that work.

The more I read of the "scientific" explanations of what NDEs are, the more I was shocked by their transparent flimsiness. And yet I also knew with chagrin that they were exactly the ones that the old "me" would have pointed to vaguely if someone had asked me to "explain" what an NDE is.

But people who weren't doctors couldn't be expected to know this. If what I'd undergone had happened to someone— anyone—else, it would have been remarkable enough. But that it had happened to me . . . Well, saying that it had happened "for a reason" made me a little uneasy. There was enough of the old doctor in me to know how outlandish—how grandiose, in fact—that sounded. But when I added up the sheer unlikelihood of all the details—and especially when I considered how precisely perfect a disease *E. coli* meningitis was for taking my cortex down, and my rapid and complete recovery from almost certain destruction—I simply had to take seriously the possibility that it really and truly *had* happened for a reason.

That only made me feel a greater sense of responsibility to tell my story right.

I had always made it a point of pride to keep up on the latest medical literature in my field, and to contribute as well when I had something of value to add. That I had been rocketed out of this world and into another one was news—genuine medical news—and now that I was back, I was not going to sell it short. Medically speaking, that I had recovered completely was a flat-out impossibility, a medical miracle. But the real story lay in where I had been, and I had a duty not just as a scientist and a profound respecter of the scientific method, but also as a healer to tell that story. A story—a true story—can heal as much as medicine can. Susanna had known that when she called me that day in my office. And I'd experienced as much myself when I'd heard back from my birth family. What had happened to me was healing news, too. What kind of a healer would I be if I didn't share it?

A little over two years after returning from coma, I visited a close friend and colleague who chairs one of the foremost academic neuroscience departments in the world. I've known John (not his real name) for decades and consider him a wonderful human being and a first-rate scientist.

I told John some of the story of my spiritual journey deep in coma, and he looked quite amazed. Not amazed at how crazy I now was, but as if he was finally making sense of something that had mystified him for a long time.

It turned out that about a year earlier, John's father was nearing the end of a five-year illness. He was incapacitated, demented, in pain, and wanted to die.

"Please," his father had begged John from his deathbed. "Give me some pills, or something. I can't go on like this."

Then suddenly his father became more cogent than he had been in two years, as he discussed some deep observations about his life and about their family. He then shifted his gaze and began talking to the air at the foot of his bed. Listening, John realized that his father was talking to his deceased mother, who had died sixty-five years before, when John's father was just a teenager. He had barely mentioned her during John's life but now was having a joyous and animated discussion with her. John could not see her but was absolutely convinced that her spirit was there, welcoming his father's spirit home.

After a few minutes of this, John's father turned back to him, a completely different look in his eye. He was smiling, and clearly very much at peace, more than John could ever remember seeing in him before.

"Go to sleep, Dad," John found himself saying. "Just let go. It's okay."

His father did just that. Closing his eyes, he drifted off with a look of complete peace on his face. Shortly thereafter, he passed on.

John felt the encounter between his father and his departed grandmother was very real, but he had not known what to do with it because, as a doctor, he knew such things were "impossible." Many others have seen that astonishing clarity of mind that often comes to demented elderly people just before they pass on, just as John had seen in his father (a phenomenon known as "terminal lucidity"). There was no neuroscientific explanation for *that*. Hearing my story seemed to give him a license he had been longing for someone to give him: the license to believe what he had seen with his own eyes—to *know* that deep and comforting truth: that our eternal spiritual self is more real than anything we perceive in this physical realm, and has a divine connection to the infinite love of the Creator.

32

A Visit to Church

There are only two ways to live your life. One is as though nothing is a miracle. The other is as if everything is.

—ALBERT EINSTEIN (1879–1955)

I didn't make it back to church until December 2008, when Holley coaxed me out to services for the second Sunday of Advent. I was still weak, still a bit off balance, still underweight. Holley and I sat in the front row. Michael Sullivan was presiding over the service that day, and he came up and asked if I felt like lighting the second candle on the Advent wreath. I didn't want to, but something told me to do it anyhow. I stood up, put my hand on the brass pole, and strode to the front of the church with unexpected ease.

My memory of my time out of the body was still naked and raw, and everywhere I turned in this place that had failed to move me much before, I saw art and heard music that brought it all right back. The pulsing bass note of a hymn echoed the rough misery of the Realm of the Earthworm's-Eye View. The stained glass windows with their clouds and angels brought to mind the celestial beauty of the Gateway. A painting of Jesus breaking bread with his disciples evoked the communion of the Core. I

2nd Chance John 3:16

shuddered as I recalled the bliss of infinite unconditional love I had known there.

At last, I understood what religion was really all about. Or at least was supposed to be about. I didn't just believe in God; I knew God. As I hobbled to the altar to take Communion, tears streamed down my cheeks.

33.

The Enigma of Consciousness

If you would be a real seeker after truth, it is necessary that at least once in your life you doubt, as far as possible, all things.

—RENÉ DESCARTES (1596–1650)

It took about two months for my full battery of neurosurgical knowledge to come back to me. Leaving aside for the moment the essentially miraculous fact that it *did* come back (there continues to be no medical precedent for my case, in which a brain under long-term attack of such a severe degree by gram-negative bacteria like *E. coli* recovers anything like its full abilities), once it had, I continued to wrestle with the fact that everything I had learned in four decades of study and work about the human brain, about the universe, and about what constitutes reality conflicted with what I'd experienced during those seven days in coma. When I fell into my coma, I was a secular doctor who had spent his entire career in some of the most prestigious research institutions in the world, trying to understand the connections between the human brain and consciousness. It wasn't that I didn't believe in consciousness. I was simply more aware than most people of the staggering mechanical unlikelihood that it existed independently—at all!

In the 1920s, the physicist Werner Heisenberg (and other founders of the science of quantum mechanics) made a discovery so strange that the world has yet to completely come to terms with it. When observing subatomic phenomena, it is impossible to completely separate the observer (that is, the scientist making the experiment) from what is being observed. In our day-to-day world, it is easy to miss this fact. We see the universe as a place full of separate objects (tables and chairs, people and planets) that occasionally interact with each other, but that nonetheless remain essentially separate. On the subatomic level, however, this universe of separate objects turns out to be a complete illusion. In the realm of the super-super-small, every object in the physical universe is intimately connected with every other object. In fact, there are really no "objects" in the world at all, only vibrations of energy, and relationships.

What that meant should have been obvious, though it wasn't to many. It was impossible to pursue the core reality of the universe without using consciousness. Far from being an unimportant by-product of physical processes (as I had thought before my experience), consciousness is not only very real—it's actually *more real* than the rest of physical existence, and most likely the basis of it all. But neither of these insights has yet been truly incorporated into science's picture of reality. Many scientists are trying to do so, but as of yet there is no unified "theory of everything" that can combine the laws of quantum mechanics with those of relativity theory in a way that begins to incorporate consciousness.

All the objects in the physical universe are made up of atoms. Atoms, in turn, are made up of protons, electrons, and neutrons. These, in turn, are (as physicists also discovered in the early years of the twentieth century) all particles. And particles are made up of . . . Well, quite frankly, physicists don't really know. But one thing we do know about particles is that each one is connected to every other one in the universe. They are all, at the deepest level, interconnected.

Before my experience out beyond, I was generally aware of all these modern scientific ideas, but they were distant and remote. In the world I lived and moved in—the world of cars and houses and operating tables and patients who did well or not depending partially on whether I operated on them successfully—these facts of subatomic physics were rarefied and removed. They might be true, but they didn't concern my daily reality.

But when I left my physical body behind, I experienced these facts directly. In fact, I feel confident in saying that, while I didn't even know the term at the time, while in the Gateway and in the Core, I was actually "doing science." Science that relied on the truest and most sophisticated tool for scientific research that we possess:

Consciousness itself.

The further I dug, the more convinced I became that my discovery wasn't just interesting or dramatic. It was *scientific*. Depending on whom you talk to, consciousness is either the greatest mystery facing scientific enquiry, or a total nonproblem. What's surprising is just how many more scientists think it's the latter. For many—maybe most—scientists, consciousness isn't really worth worrying about because it is just a by-product of physical processes. Many scientists go further, saying that not only is consciousness a secondary phenomenon, but that in addition, it's not even *real*.

Many leaders in the neuroscience of consciousness and the philosophy of mind, however, would beg to differ. Over the last few decades, they have come to recognize the "hard problem of consciousness." Although the idea had been coalescing for decades, it was David Chalmers who defined it in his brilliant

1996 book, *The Conscious Mind*. The hard problem concerns the very existence of conscious experience and can be distilled into these questions:

How does consciousness arise out of the functioning of the human brain?

How is it related to the behavior that it accompanies?

How does the perceived world relate to the real world?

The hard problem is so hard to resolve that some thinkers have said the answer lies outside of "science" altogether. But that it lies outside the bounds of current science in no way belittles the phenomenon of consciousness—in fact, it is a clue as to its unfathomably profound role in the universe.

The ascendance of the scientific method based solely in the physical realm over the past four hundred years presents a major problem: we have lost touch with the deep mystery at the center of existence—our consciousness. It was (under different names and expressed through different world-views) something known well and held close by pre-modern religions, but it was lost to our secular Western culture as we became increasingly enamored with the power of modern science and technology.

For all of the successes of Western civilization, the world has paid a dear price in terms of the most crucial component of existence—our human spirit. The shadow side of high technology—modern warfare and thoughtless homicide and suicide, urban blight, ecological mayhem, cataclysmic climate change, polarization of economic resources—is bad enough. Much worse, our focus on exponential progress in science and technology has left many of us relatively bereft in the realm of meaning and joy, and of knowing how our lives fit into the grand scheme of existence for all eternity.

Questions concerning the soul and afterlife, reincarnation,

God, and Heaven proved difficult to answer through conventional scientific means, which implied that they might not exist. Likewise, extended consciousness phenomena, such as remote viewing, extrasensory perception, psychokinesis, clairvoyance, telepathy, and precognition, have seemed stubbornly resistant to comprehend through "standard" scientific investigations. Before my coma, I doubted their veracity, mainly because I had never experienced them at a deep level, and because they could not be readily explained by my simplistic scientific view of the world.

Like many other scientific skeptics, I refused to even review the data relevant to the questions concerning these phenomena. I prejudged the data, and those providing it, because my limited perspective failed to provide the foggiest notion of how such things might actually happen. Those who assert that there is no evidence for phenomena indicative of extended consciousness, in spite of overwhelming evidence to the contrary, are willfully ignorant. They believe they know the truth without needing to look at the facts.

For those still stuck in the trap of scientific skepticism, I recommend the book *Irreducible Mind: Toward a Psychology for the 21st Century,* published in 2007. The evidence for out-of-body consciousness is well presented in this rigorous scientific analysis. *Irreducible Mind* is a landmark opus from a highly reputable group, the Division of Perceptual Studies, based at the University of Virginia. The authors provide an exhaustive review of the relevant data, and the conclusion is inescapable: these phenomena are real, and we must try to understand their nature if we want to comprehend the reality of our existence.

We have been seduced into thinking that the scientific world view is fast approaching a Theory of Everything (or TOE), which would not seem to leave much room for our soul, or spirit, or for Heaven, and God. My journey deep into coma, outside of this lowly physical realm and into the loftiest dwelling place of the almighty Creator, revealed the indescribably immense chasm between our human knowledge and the awe-inspiring realm of God.

Each one of us is more familiar with consciousness than we are with anything else, and yet we understand far more about the rest of the universe than we do about the mechanism of consciousness. It is *so* close to home that it is almost forever beyond our grasp. There is nothing about the physics of the material world (quarks, electrons, photons, atoms, etc.), and specifically the intricate structure of the brain, that gives the slightest clue as to the mechanism of consciousness.

In fact, the greatest clue to the reality of the spiritual realm is this *profound mystery* of our conscious existence. This is a far more mysterious revelation than physicists or neuroscientists have shown themselves capable of dealing with, and their failure to do so has left the intimate relationship between consciousness and quantum mechanics—and thus physical reality—obscured.

To truly study the universe on a deep level, we must acknowledge the fundamental role of consciousness in painting reality. Experiments in quantum mechanics shocked those brilliant fathers of the field, many of whom (Werner Heisenberg, Wolfgang Pauli, Niels Bohr, Erwin Schrödinger, Sir James Jeans, to name a few) turned to the mystical worldview seeking answers. They realized it was impossible to separate the experimenter from the experiment, and to explain reality without consciousness. What I discovered out beyond is the indescribable immensity and complexity of the universe, and that *consciousness* is the basis of all that exists. I was so totally connected to it that there was often no real differentiation between "me" and the world I was moving through. If I had to summarize all this, I would say first, that the universe is much larger than it appears to be if we only look at its immediately visible parts. (This isn't much of a revolutionary insight actually, as conventional science acknowledges that 96 percent of the universe is made up of "dark matter and energy." What are these dark entities?* No one yet knows. But what made my experience unusual was the jolting immediacy with which I experienced the basic role of consciousness, or spirit. It wasn't theory when I learned this up there, but a fact, overwhelming and immediate as a blast of arctic air in the face.) Second: We—each of us—are intricately, irremovably connected to the larger universe. It is our true home, and thinking that this physical world is all that matters is like shutting oneself up in a small closet and imagining that there is nothing else out beyond it. And third: the crucial power of *belief* in facilitating "mind-over-matter." I was often bemused as a medical student over the confounding power of the placebo effect—that medical studies had to overcome the 30 percent or so benefit that was attributed to a patient's believing that he was receiving medicine that would help him, even if it was simply an inert substance. Instead of seeing the underlying power of belief, and how it influenced our health, the medical profession saw the glass as "half-empty"—that the placebo effect was an obstacle to the demonstration of a treatment.

At the heart of the enigma of quantum mechanics lies the

---

* Seventy percent is "dark energy," that most mysterious force discovered by astronomers in the mid-1990s as they found incontrovertible proof based on Type Ia supernovas that for the last five billion years the universe has been falling *up*—that the expansion of all of space is *accelerating*. Another 26 percent is "dark matter," the anomalous "excess" gravity revealed over the last few decades in the rotation of galaxies and galactic clusters. Explanations will be made, but the mysteries beyond will never end.

falsehood of our notion of locality in space and time. The rest of the universe—that is, the vast majority of it—isn't actually distant from us in space. Yes, physical space seems real, but it is limited as well. The entire length and height of the physical universe is as nothing to the spiritual realm from which it has risen—the realm of consciousness (which some might refer to as "the life force").

This other, vastly grander universe isn't "far away" at all. In fact, it's right here—right here where I am, typing this sentence, and right there where you are, reading it. It's not far away physically, but simply exists on a different frequency. It's right here, right now, but we're unaware of it because we are for the most part closed to those frequencies on which it manifests. We live in the dimensions of familiar space and time, hemmed in by the peculiar limitations of our sensory organs and by our perceptual scaling within the spectrum from subatomic quantum up through the entire universe. Those dimensions, while they have many things going for them, also shut us out from the other dimensions that exist as well.

The ancient Greeks discovered all of this long ago, and I was only discovering for myself what they'd already hit upon: Like understands like. The universe is so constructed that to truly understand any part of its many dimensions and levels, *you have to become a part of that dimension*. Or, stated a little more accurately, you have to open yourself to an identity with that part of the universe that you already possess, but which you may not have been conscious of.

The universe has no beginning or end, and God is entirely present within every particle of it. Much—in fact, most—of what people have had to say about God and the higher spiritual worlds has involved bringing them down to our level, rather than elevating our perceptions up to theirs. We taint, with our insufficient descriptions, their truly awesome nature.

But though it never began and will never end, the universe does have punctuation marks, the purpose of which is to bring beings into existence and allow them to participate in the glory of God. The Big Bang that created our universe was one of these creative "punctuation marks." Om's view was from outside, encompassing all of Om's Creation and beyond even my higher-dimensional field of view. Here, to see was to know. There was no distinction between experiencing something and my understanding it.

"I was blind, but now I see," now took on a new meaning as I understood just how blind to the full nature of the spiritual universe we are on earth—especially people like I had been, who had believed that matter was the core reality, and that all else—thought, consciousness, ideas, emotions, spirit—were simply productions of it.

This revelation inspired me greatly, because it allowed me to see the staggering heights of communion and understanding that lie ahead for us all, when each of us leaves the limitations of our physical body and brain behind.

Humor. Irony. Pathos. I had always thought these were qualities we humans developed to cope with this so often painful and unfair world. And they are. But in addition to being consolations, these qualities are *recognitions*—brief, flashing, but all-important—of the fact that whatever our struggles and sufferings in the present world are, they can't truly touch the larger, eternal beings we in truth are. Laughter and irony are at heart reminders that we are not prisoners in this world, but voyagers through it.

Another aspect of the good news is that you don't have to almost die to glimpse behind the veil—but you must do the work. Learning about that realm from books and presentations is a start—but at the end of the day, we each have to go deep into our own consciousness, through prayer or meditation, to access these truths.

Meditation comes in many different forms. The most useful for me since my coma has been that developed by Robert A. Monroe, founder of the Monroe Institute in Faber, Virginia. Their freedom from any dogmatic philosophy offers a distinct advantage. The only dogma associated with Monroe's system of meditative exercises is: *I am more than my physical body.* This simple acknowledgment has profound implications.

Robert Monroe was a successful radio program producer in the 1950s in New York. In the process of investigating the use of audio recordings as a sleep-learning technique, he began to have out-of-body experiences. His detailed research over more than four decades has resulted in a powerful system to enhance deep conscious exploration based on an audio technology he developed known as "Hemi-Sync."

Hemi-Sync can heighten selective awareness and performance through creation of a relaxed state. Hemi-Sync offers much more than this, however—enhanced states of consciousness allow access to alternate perceptual modes, including deep meditation and mystical states. Hemi-Sync involves the physics of resonant entrainment of brain waves, their relationship to the perceptual and behavioral psychology of consciousness, and to the fundamental physiology of the brain-mind and consciousness.

Hemi-Sync uses specific patterns of stereo sound waves (of slightly different frequencies in each ear) to induce synchronized brain wave activity. These "binaural beats" are generated at a frequency that is the arithmetic difference between the two signal frequencies. By using an ancient but highly accurate timing system in the brainstem that normally enables localization of sound sources in the horizontal plane around the head, these binaural beats can entrain the adjacent Reticular Activating System, which provides steady timing signals to the thalamus and cortex enabling consciousness. These signals generate brain wave synchrony in the range of 1 to 25 hertz (Hz, or cycles per second), including the crucial region below the normal threshold for human hearing (20 Hz). This lowest range is associated with brain waves in the delta (< 4 Hz, normally found in deep dreamless sleep), theta (4 to 7 Hz, seen in deep meditation and relaxation, and in non-REM sleep), and alpha ranges (7 to 13 Hz, characteristic of REM or dream sleep, drowsiness at the borders of sleep, and awakened relaxation).

In my journey of understanding after my coma, Hemi-Sync potentially offered a means of inactivating the filtering function of the physical brain by globally synchronizing my neocortical electrical activity, just as my meningitis might have done, to liberate my out-of-body consciousness. I believe Hemi-Sync has enabled me to return to a realm similar to that which I visited deep in coma, but without having to be deathly ill. But just as in my dreams of flying as a child, this is very much a process of *allowing* the journey to unfold—if I try to force it, to over-*think* it, or embrace the process too much, it doesn't work.

To use the word *all-knowing* feels inappropriate, because the awe and creative power I witnessed was beyond naming. I realized that the proscriptions of some religions against naming God or depicting divine prophets did indeed have an intuitive correctness to them, because God's reality is in truth so completely beyond any of our human attempts at capturing God in words or pictures while here on earth.

Just as my awareness was both individual yet at the same time completely unified with the universe, so also did the boundaries of what I experienced as my "self" at times contract, and at other times expand to include all that exists throughout eternity. The blurring of the boundary between my awareness and the realm around me went so far at times that I *became* the entire universe. Another way of putting this would be to say that I momentarily saw an identity with the universe, which had been there all the time, but that I had just been blind to up till then.

An analogy I often use to demonstrate my consciousness at that deepest level is that of a hen's egg. While in the Core, even when I became one with the Orb of light and the entire higher-dimensional universe throughout all eternity, and was intimately one with God, I sensed strongly that the creative, primordial (prime mover) aspect of God was the shell around the egg's contents, intimately associated throughout (as our consciousness is a direct extension of the Divine), yet forever beyond the capability of absolute identification with the consciousness of the created. Even as my consciousness became identical with all and eternity, I sensed that I could not become entirely one with the creative, originating driver of all that is. At the heart of the most infinite oneness, there was still that duality. It is possible that such apparent duality is simply the result of trying to bring such awareness back into this realm.

I never heard Om's voice directly, nor saw Om's face. It was as if Om spoke to me through thoughts that were like wave-walls rolling through me, rocking everything around me and showing that there is a deeper fabric of existence—a fabric that all of us are always part of, but which we're generally not conscious of.

So I was communicating directly with God? Absolutely. Expressed that way, it sounds grandiose. But when it was happening, it didn't feel that way. Instead, I felt like I was doing what every soul is able to do when they leave their bodies, and what we can all do right now through various methods of prayer or deep meditation. Communicating with God is the most extraordinary experience imaginable, yet at the same time it's the most natural one of all, because God is present in us at all times. Omniscient, omnipotent, personal—and loving us without conditions. We are connected as One through our divine link with God.

34.

A Final Dilemma

*I must be willing to give up what I am
in order to become what I will be.*

—Albert Einstein (1879–1955)

Einstein was one of my early scientific idols and the above quote of his had always been one of my favorites. But I now understood what those words actually meant. Crazy as I knew it sounded every time I told my story to one of my scientific colleagues—as I could see in their glazed or perturbed expressions—I knew I was telling them something that had genuine scientific validity. And that it opened the door to a whole new world—a whole new universe—of scientific comprehension. Observation that honored consciousness itself as the single greatest entity in all of existence.

But one common event in NDEs had not happened with me. Or, more accurately, there was a small group of experiences I had not undergone, and all of these clustered around one fact:

While out, I had not remembered my earthly identity.

Though no two NDEs are exactly alike, I'd discovered early on in my reading that there is a very consistent list of typical features that many contain. One of these is a meeting with one or more deceased people that the NDE subject had known in life. I had met no one I'd known in life. But that part didn't bother me so much, as I'd already discovered that my forgetting of my earthly identity had allowed me to move further "in" than many NDE subjects do. There was certainly nothing to complain about in that. What did bother me was that there was one person I would have deeply loved to have met. My dad had died four years before I entered coma. Given that he knew how I felt I had failed to measure up to his standards during those lost years of mine, why had he not been there to tell me it was okay? For comfort was, indeed, what the NDE subject's friends or family who greeted them were most often intent on conveying. I longed for that comfort. And yet I hadn't received it.

It wasn't that I hadn't received any words of comfort at all, of course. I had, from the Girl on the Butterfly Wing. But wonderful and angelic as this girl was, she was *no one I knew*. Having seen her every time I entered that idyllic valley on the wing of a butterfly, I remembered her face perfectly—so much so that I knew I had never met her in my life, at least my life on earth. And in NDEs it was often the meeting with a known earthly friend or relation that sealed the deal for the people who had undergone these experiences.

Try as I did to brush it off, this fact introduced an element of doubt into my thoughts on what it all meant. It wasn't that I doubted what had happened to me. That was impossible, and I'd have just as soon doubted my marriage to Holley or my love for my kids. But the fact that I had traveled to the beyond without meeting my father, and met my beautiful companion on the butterfly wing, whom I didn't know, still troubled me. Given the intensely emotional nature of my relationship to my family, my feelings of lack of worth because I had been given away, why hadn't that all-important message—that I was loved, that I would never be thrown away—been delivered by someone I knew? Someone like . . . my dad?

For in fact, "thrown away" was, on a deep level, how I had indeed felt all through my life—in spite of all the best efforts of my family to heal that feeling through their love. My Dad had often told me not to be overly concerned about whatever had happened to me before he and Mom had picked me up at the children's home. "You wouldn't remember anything that happened to you that early anyhow," he'd said. And in that he'd been wrong. My NDE had convinced me that there is a secret part of ourselves that is recording every last aspect of our earthly lives, and that this recording process commences at the very, very beginning. So on a precognitive, preverbal level, I'd known all through my life that I'd been given away, and on a deep level I was still struggling to forgive that fact.

As long as this question remained open, there would remain a dismissive voice. One that told me, insistently and even deviously, that for all the perfection and wonder of my NDE, something had been missing, had been "off" about it.

In essence, a part of me still doubted the authenticity of my astonishingly real deep-coma experience, and thus of the true existence of that entire realm. To that part of me, it continued to "not make sense" from a scientific standpoint. And that small but insistent voice of doubt began to threaten the whole new worldview I was slowly building.

35.

The Photograph

Gratitude is not only the greatest of virtues,
but the parent of all others.

—CICERO (106–43 BCE)

Four months after my departure from the hospital, my birth family sister Kathy finally got around to sending me a photo of my birth sister Betsy. I was up in our bedroom, where my odyssey all began, when I opened the oversized envelope and pulled out a framed glossy color photo of the sister I had never known. She was standing, I would later find out, near the dock ing pier of the Balboa Island Ferry near her home in Southern California, a beautiful West Coast sunset in the background. She had long brown hair and deep blue eyes, and her smile, radiating love and kindness, seemed to go right through me, making my heart both swell and ache at the same time.

Kathy had affixed a poem over the photo. It was written by David M. Romano in 1993, and was called "When Tomorrow Starts Without Me."

When tomorrow starts without me,
And I'm not there to see,
If the sun should rise and find your eyes
All filled with tears for me;

I wish so much you wouldn't cry
The way you did today,
While thinking of the many things,
We didn't get to say.
I know how much you love me,
As much as I love you,
And each time you think of me,
I know you'll miss me too;
But when tomorrow starts without me,
Please try to understand,
That an angel came and called my name,
And took me by the hand,
And said my place was ready,
In heaven far above
And that I'd have to leave behind
All those I dearly love.
But as I turned to walk away,
A tear fell from my eye
For all my life, I'd always thought,
I didn't want to die.
I had so much to live for,
So much left yet to do,
It seemed almost impossible,
That I was leaving you.

I thought of all the yesterdays,
The good ones and the bad,
The thought of all the love we shared,
And all the fun we had.
If I could relive yesterday
Just even for a while,

I'd say good-bye and kiss you
And maybe see you smile.
But then I fully realized
That this could never be,
For emptiness and memories,
Would take the place of me.
And when I thought of worldly things
I might miss come tomorrow,
I thought of you, and when I did
My heart was filled with sorrow.
But when I walked through heaven's gates
I felt so much at home
When God looked down and smiled at me,
From His great golden throne,
He said, "This is eternity,
And all I've promised you.
Today your life on earth is past
But here it starts anew.
I promise no tomorrow,
But today will always last,
And since each day's the same way,
There's no longing for the past.
You have been so faithful,
So trusting and so true.
Though there were times
You did some things
You knew you shouldn't do.
But you have been forgiven
And now at last you're free.
So won't you come and take my hand
And share my life with me?"

So when tomorrow starts without me,
Don't think we're far apart,
For every time you think of me,
I'm right here, in your heart.

My eyes were misting as I put the picture carefully up on the dresser and continued to stare at it. She looked so strangely, hauntingly familiar. But of course, she *would* look that way. We were blood relations and had shared more DNA than any other people on the planet with the exception of my other two biological siblings. Whether we'd ever met or not, Betsy and I were deeply connected.

The next morning, I was in our bedroom reading more of the Elisabeth Kübler-Ross book *On Life After Death* when I came to a story about a twelve-year-old girl who underwent an NDE and at first didn't tell her parents about it. Finally, however, she could no longer keep it to herself and confided in her father. She told him about traveling to an incredible landscape full of love and beauty, and how she met and was comforted by her brother.

"The only problem," the girl told her father, "is that I don't have a brother."

Tears filled her father's eyes. He told the girl about the brother she did indeed have, but who had died just three months before she was born.

I stopped reading. For a moment I went into a strange, dazed space, not really thinking or not thinking, just . . . absorbing something. Some thought that was right on the edge of my consciousness but hadn't quite broken through.

Then my eyes traveled over to the bureau, and the photo that Kathy had sent me. The photo of the sister I had never known. Whom I knew only through the stories that my birth family had related of what a hugely kind, wonderfully caring person she had been. A person, they had often said, who was so kind she was practically an angel.

Without the powder blue and indigo dress, without the heavenly light of the Gateway around her as she sat on the beautiful butterfly wing, she wasn't easy to recognize at first. But that was only natural. I had seen her heavenly self—the one that lived above and beyond this earthly realm, with all its tragedies and cares.

But now there was no mistaking her, no mistaking the loving smile, the confident and infinitely comforting look, the sparkling blue eyes.

It was she.

For an instant, the worlds met. My world here on earth, where I was a doctor and father and a husband. And that world out there—a world so vast that as you journeyed in it you could lose your very sense of your earthly self and become a pure part of the cosmos, the God-soaked and love-filled darkness.

In that one moment, in the bedroom of our house, on a rainy Tuesday morning, the higher and the lower worlds met. Seeing that photo made me feel a little like the boy in the fairy tale who travels to the other world and then returns, only to find that it was all a dream—until he looks in his pocket and finds a scintillating handful of magical earth from the realms beyond.

As much as I'd tried to deny it, for weeks now a fight had been going on inside me. A fight between the part of my mind that had been out there beyond the body, and the doctor—the healer who had pledged himself to science. I looked into the face of my sister, my angel, and I knew—knew completely—that the two people I had been in the last few months, since coming back, were indeed one. I needed to completely embrace my role as a doctor, as a scientist and healer, and as the subject of a very unlikely, very real, very important journey into the Divine itself. It was important not because of me, but because of the fantastically, deal-breakingly convincing details behind it. My NDE had healed my fragmented soul. It had let me know that I had always been loved, and it also showed me that absolutely everyone else in the universe is loved, too. And it had done so while placing my physical body into a state that, by medical science's current terms, should have made it impossible for me to have experienced *anything*.

I know there will be people who will seek to invalidate my experience anyhow, and many who will discount it out of court, because of a refusal to believe that what I underwent could possibly be "scientific"—could possibly by anything more than a crazy, feverish dream.

But I know better. And both for the sake of those here on earth and those I met beyond this realm, I see it as my duty— both as a scientist and hence a seeker of truth, and as a doctor devoted to helping people—to make it known to as many people as I can that what I underwent is true, and real, and of stunning importance. Not just to me, but to all of us.

Not only was my journey about love, but it was also about who we are and how connected we all are—the very meaning of all existence. I learned who I was up there, and when I came back, I realized that the last broken strands of who I am down here were sewn up.

You are loved. Those words are what I needed to hear as an orphan, as a child who'd been given away. But it's also what every one of us in this materialistic age needs to hear as well, because in terms of who we really are, where we really came from, and where we're really going, we all feel (wrongly) like orphans.

Without recovering that memory of our larger connectedness, and of the unconditional love of our Creator, we will always feel lost here on earth.

So here I am. I'm still a scientist, I'm still a doctor, and as such I have two essential duties: to honor truth and to help heal. That means telling my story. A story that as time passes I feel certain happened for a reason. Not because I'm anyone special. It's just that with me, two events occurred in unison and concurrence, and together they break the back of the last efforts of reductive science to tell the world that the material realm is all that exists, and that consciousness, or spirit—yours and mine—is not the great and central mystery of the universe.

I'm living proof.

Eternea

My near-death experience inspired me to help make the world a better place for all, and Eternea is the vehicle to enable that fundamental change. Eternea is a nonprofit publicly supported charity I cofounded with my friend and colleague, John R. Audette. Eternea represents a passionate effort to serve the greater good by helping to create the best possible future for earth and its inhabitants.

Eternea's mission is to advance research, education, and applied programs concerning spiritually transformative experiences, as well as the physics of consciousness and the interactive relationship between consciousness and physical reality (e.g., matter and energy). It is an organized effort to apply in practical ways not only the insights gained from near-death experiences, but also to serve as a repository for all manner of spiritually transformative experiences.

Please visit www.Eternea.org to further your own spiritual awakening or to share your own personal story about a spiritually transformative experience you may have had (or if you are grieving from the loss of a loved one, or if you are facing a terminal illness or a loved one is). Eternea will also provide a valuable resource for scientists, academicians, researchers, theologians, and members of the clergy who are interested in this field of study.

Eben Alexander, M.D.
Lynchburg, Virginia
July 10, 2012

Acknowledgments

I wish to especially acknowledge my dear family for suffering through the hardest part of this experience, while I was in coma. To Holley, my wife of thirty-one years, and our wonderful sons, Eben IV and Bond, who all played central roles in bringing me back, and in helping me comprehend my experience. Additional dear family and friends to thank include my beloved parents Betty and Eben Alexander, Jr., and my sisters Jean, Betsy, and Phyllis, who all participated in a pact (with Holley, Bond, and Eben IV) to hold my hand 24/7 while I was in coma, assuring that I always felt the touch of their love. Betsy and Phyllis did yeoman's work in spending nights with me during my full-blown ICU psychosis (when I couldn't sleep at all, *ever*) and in those first very tenuous days and nights after I went to the Neuroscience Step-down Unit. Peggy Daly (Holley's sister) and Sylvia White (Holley's friend of thirty years) were also part of the constant vigil in my room on the ICU. I never could have returned without their individual loving efforts to bring me back to this world. To Dayton and Jack Slye, who did without their mother, Phyllis, while she was with me. Holley, Eben IV, Mom, and Phyllis also helped in editing and critiquing my story.

My heaven-sent birth family, and especially my departed sister, also named Betsy, whom I never met in this world.

My blessed and capable doctors at Lynchburg General Hospital (LGH), especially Drs. Scott Wade, Robert Brennan, Laura Potter, Michael Milam, Charlie Joseph, Sarah and Tim Hellewell, and many more.

The extraordinary nurses and staff at LGH: Rhae Newbill, Lisa Flowers, Dana Andrews, Martha Vesterlund, Deanna Tomlin, Valerie Walters, Janice Sonowski, Molly Mannis, Diane Newman, Joanne Robinson, Janet Phillips, Christina Costello, Larry Bowen, Robin Price, Amanda Decoursey, Brooke Reynolds, and Erica Stalkner. I was comatose and had to get names from my family, so forgive me if you were there and I have omitted your name.

Critical to my return were Michael Sullivan and Susan Reintjes.

John Audette, Raymond Moody, Bill Guggenheim, and Ken Ring, pioneers in the near-death community, whose influence on me has been immeasurable (not to mention Bill's excellent editorial assistance).

Other thought leaders of the "Virginia Consciousness" movement, including Drs. Bruce Greyson, Ed Kelly, Emily Williams Kelly, Jim Tucker, Ross Dunseath, and Bob Van de Castle.

My God-sent literary agent, Gail Ross, and her wonderful associates, Howard Yoon and others at the Ross Yoon Agency.

Ptolemy Tompkins for his scholarly contributions from unparalleled insight into several millennia of literature on the afterlife, and for his superb editorial and writing skills, used to weave my experience into this book, truly doing it the justice it deserved.

Priscilla Painton, vice president and executive editor, and Jonathan Karp, executive vice president and publisher at Simon & Schuster, for their extraordinary vision and passion to make this world a far better place.

Marvin and Terre Hamlisch, wonderful friends whose enthusiasm and passionate interest carried me through at a critical time.

Terri Beavers and Margaretta McIlvaine for their brilliant bridging of healing and spirituality.

Karen Newell for sharing explorations into deep conscious states and teaching how to "Be the love that you are," and to the other miracle workers at the Monroe Institute in Faber, Virginia, especially Robert Monroe for pursuing what *is*, and not just what *should be;* Carol Sabick de la Herran and Karen Malik, who sought me out; and Paul Rademacher and Skip Atwater, who welcomed me into that loving community in the ethereal high mountain meadows in central Virginia. Also, to Kevin Kossi, Patty Avalon, Penny Holmes, Joe and Nancy "Scooter" McMoneagle, Scott Taylor, Cindy Johnston, Amy Hardie, Loris Adams, and all of my fellow Gateway Voyagers at the Monroe Institute in February 2011, my facilitators (Charleene Nicely, Rob Sandstrom, and Andrea Berger) and fellow Lifeline participants (and facilitators Franceen King and Joe Gallenberger) in July 2011.

My good friends and critics, Jay Gainsboro, Judson Newbern, Dr. Allan Hamilton, and Kitch Carter, who read early versions of this manuscript and sensed my frustration in synthesizing my spiritual experience with neuroscience. Judson and Allan were critical in helping me appreciate the true power of my experience from the viewpoint of the scientist/skeptic, and Jay the same from the standpoint of the scientist/mystic.

Fellow explorers of deep consciousness and the Oneness, including Elke Siller Macartney and Jim Macartney.

My fellow near-death experiencers Andrea Curewitz, for her excellent editorial advice, and Carolyn Tyler, for her soulful guidance in my understanding.

Blitz and Heidi James, Susan Carrington, Mary Horner, Mimi Sykes, and Nancy Clark, whose courage and faith in the face of unfathomable loss helped me to appreciate my gift.

Janet Sussman, Martha Harbison, Shobhan (Rick) and Danna Faulds, Sandra Glickman, and Sharif Abdullah, fellow travelers whom I first met on 11/11/11, gathered together to share our seven optimistic visions of a brilliant conscious future for all of humanity.

Numerous additional people to thank include the many friends whose acts during that most difficult time, and whose thoughtful comments and observations have helped my family and guided the telling of my story: Judy and Dickie Stowers, Susan Carrington, Jackie and Dr. Ron Hill, Drs. Mac McCrary and George Hurt, Joanna and Dr. Walter Beverly, Catherine and Wesley Robinson, Bill and Patty Wilson, DeWitt and Jeff Kierstead, Toby Beavers, Mike and Linda Milam, Heidi Baldwin, Mary Brockman, Karen and George Lupton, Norm and Paige Darden, Geisel and Kevin Nye, Joe and Betty Mullen, Buster and Lynn Walker, Susan Whitehead, Jeff Horsley, Clara Bell, Courtney and Johnny Alford, Gilson and Dodge Lincoln, Liz Smith, Sophia Cody, Lone Jensen, Suzanne and Steve Johnson, Copey Hanes, Bob and Stephanie Sullivan, Diane and Todd Vie, Colby Proffitt, the Taylor, Reams, Tatom, Heppner, Sullivan, and Moore families, and so many others.

My gratitude, most especially to God, is unbounded.

Reading List

Atwater, F. Holmes. *Captain of My Ship, Master of My Soul.* Charlottesville, VA: Hampton Roads, 2001.

Atwater, P. M. H. *Near-Death Experiences: The Rest of the Story.* Charlottesville, VA: Hampton Roads, 2011.

Bache, Christopher. *Dark Night, Early Dawn: Steps to a Deeper Ecology of Mind.* Albany, NY: State University of New York Press, 2000.

Buhlman, William. *The Secret of the Soul: Using Out-of-Body Experiences to Understand Our True Nature.* New York: HarperCollins, 2001.

Callanan, Maggie, and Patricia Kelley. *Final Gifts: Understanding the Special Awareness, Needs, and Communications of the Dying.* New York: Poseidon Press, 1992.

Carhart-Harris, RL, *et alia*, "Neural correlates of the psychedelic state determined by fMRI studies with psilocybin," *Proc. Nat. Acad Of Sciences* 109, no. 6 (Feb. 2012): 2138–2143.

Carter, Chris. *Science and the Near-Death Experience: How Consciousness Survives Death.* Rochester, VT: Inner Traditions, 2010.

Chalmers, David J. *The Conscious Mind: In Search of a Fundamental Theory.* Oxford: Oxford University Press, 1996.

Churchland, Paul M. *The Engine of Reason, the Seat of the Soul.* Cambridge, MA: MIT Press, 1995.

Collins, Francis S. *The Language of God: A Scientist Presents Evidence for Belief.* New York: Simon & Schuster, 2006.

Conway, John, and Simon Kochen. "The free will theorem." *Foundations of Physics* (Springer Netherlands) 36, no. 10 (2006): 1441–73.

———. "The strong free will theorem." *Notices of the AMS* 56, no. 2 (2009): 226–32.

Dalai Lama (His Holiness the Dalai Lama). *The Universe in a Single Atom: The Convergence of Science and Spirituality.* New York: Broadway Books, 2005.

Davies, Paul. *The Mind of God: The Scientific Basis for a Rational World.* New York: Simon & Schuster, 1992.

D'Souza, Dinesh. *Life After Death: The Evidence.* Washington, DC: Regnery, Inc., 2009.

Dupré, Louis, and James A. Wiseman. *Light from Light: An Anthology of Christian Mysticism.* Mahwah, NJ: Paulist Press, 2001.

Eadie, Betty J. *Embraced by the Light.* Placerville, CA: Gold Leaf Press, 1992.

Edelman, Gerald M., and Giulio Tononi. *A Universe of Consciousness.* New York: Basic Books, 2000.

Fox, Matthew, and Rupert Sheldrake. *The Physics of Angels: Exploring the Realm Where Science and Spirit Meet.* New York: HarperCollins, 1996.

Fredrickson, Barbara. *Positivity.* New York: Crown, 2009.

Guggenheim, Bill and Judy Guggenheim. *Hello from Heaven!* New York, NY: Bantam Books, 1995.

Hagerty, Barbara Bradley. *Fingerprints of God.* New York: Riverhead Hardcover, 2009.

Haggard, P, and M Eimer. "On the relation between brain potentials and conscious awareness." *Experimental Brain Research* 126 (1999): 128–33.

Hamilton, Allan J. *The Scalpel and the Soul.* New York: Penguin Group, 2008.

Hofstadter, Douglas R. *Gödel, Escher, Bach: An Eternal Golden Braid.* New York: Basic Books, 1979.

Holden, Janice Miner, Bruce Greyson, and Debbie James., eds. *The Handbook of Near-Death Experiences: Thirty Years of Investigation.* Santa Barbara, CA: Praeger, 2009.

Houshmand, Zara, Robert B. Livingston, and B. Alan Wallace., eds. *Consciousness at the Crossroads: Conversations with the Dalai Lama on Brain Science and Buddhism.* Ithaca, NY: Snow Lion, 1999.

Jahn, Robert G., and Brenda J. Dunne. *Margins of Reality: The Role of Consciousness in the Physical World.* New York: Harcourt Brace Jovanovich, 1987.

Jampolsky, Gerald G. *Love Is Letting Go of Fear.* Berkeley, CA: Celestial Arts, 2004.

Jensen, Lone. *Gifts of Grace: A Gathering of Personal Encounters with the Virgin Mary.* New York: HarperCollins, 1995.

Johnson, Timothy. *Finding God in the Questions: A Personal Journey.* Downers Grove, IL: InterVarsity Press, 2004.

Kauffman, Stuart A. *At Home in the Universe: The Search for the Laws of Self-Organization and Complexity.* New York: Oxford University Press, 1995.

Kelly, Edward F., Emily Williams Kelly, Adam Crabtree, Alan Gauld, Michael Grosso, and Bruce Greyson. *Irreducible Mind: Toward a Psychology for the 21st Century.* Lanham, MD: Rowman & Littlefield, 2007.

Koch, C., and K. Hepp. "Quantum mechanics and higher brain functions: Lessons from quantum computation and neurobiology." *Nature* 440 (2006): 611–12.

Kübler-Ross, Elisabeth. *On Life After Death.* Berkeley, CA: Ten Speed Press, 1991.

LaBerge, Stephen, and Howard Rheingold. *Exploring the World of Lucid Dreaming.* New York: Ballantine Books, 1990.

Lau, HC, R. D. Rogers, P. Haggard, and R. E. Passingham. "Attention to intention." *Science* 303 (2004): 1208–10.

Laureys, S. "The neural correlate of (un)awareness: Lessons from the vegetative state." "Trends in Cognitive Science," in *Cognitive Science* 9 (2005): 556–59.

Libet, B, C. A. Gleason, E. W. Wright, and D. K. Pearl. "Time of conscious intention to act in relation to onset of cerebral activity (readiness-potential): The unconscious initiation of a freely voluntary act." *Brain* 106 (1983): 623–42.

Libet, Benjamin. *Mind Time: The Temporal Factor in Consciousness.* Cambridge, MA: Harvard University Press, 2004.

Llinás, Rodolfo R. *I of the Vortex: From Neurons to Self.* Cambridge, MA: MIT Press, 2001.

Lockwood, Michael. *Mind, Brain & the Quantum: The Compound 'I'.* Oxford: Basil Blackwell, 1989.

Long, Jeffrey, and Paul Perry. *Evidence of the Afterlife: The Science of Near-Death Experiences.* New York: HarperCollins, 2010.

McMoneagle, Joseph. *Mind Trek: Exploring Consciousness, Time, and Space Through Remote Viewing.* Charlottesville, VA: Hampton Roads, 1993.

———. *Remote Viewing Secrets: A Handbook.* Charlottesville, VA: Hampton Roads, 2000.

Mendoza, Marilyn A. *We Do Not Die Alone: "Jesus Is Coming to Get Me in a White Pickup Truck."* Duluth, GA: I CAN, 2008.

Monroe, Robert A. *Far Journeys.* New York: Doubleday, 1985.

———. *Journeys Out of the Body.* New York: Doubleday, 1971.

———. *Ultimate Journey.* New York: Doubleday, 1994.

Moody, Raymond A., Jr. *Life After Life: The Investigation of a Phenomenon—Survival of Bodily Death.* New York: HarperCollins, 2001.

Moody, Raymond, Jr., and Paul Perry. *Glimpses of Eternity: Sharing a Loved One's Passage from this Life to the Next.* New York: Guideposts, 2010.

Moorjani, Anita. *Dying to Be Me: My Journey from Cancer, to Near Death, to True Healing.* Carlsbad, CA: Hay House, Inc., 2012.

Morinis, E. Alan. *Everyday Holiness: The Jewish Spiritual Path of Mussar.* Boston: Shambhala, 2007.

Mountcastle, Vernon. "An Organizing Principle for Cerebral Functions: The Unit Model and the Distributed System." In *The Mindful Brain,* edited by Gerald M. Edelman and Vernon Mountcastle, pp. 7–50. Cambridge, MA: MIT Press, 1978.

Murphy, Nancey, Robert J. Russell, and William R. Stoeger., eds. *Physics and Cosmology—Scientific Perspectives on the Problem of Natural Evil.* Notre Dame, IN: Vatican Observatory and Center for Theology and the Natural Sciences, 2007.

Neihardt, John G. *Black Elk Speaks: Being the Life Story of a Holy Man of the Oglala Sioux.* Albany: State University of New York Press, 2008.

Nelson, Kevin. *The Spiritual Doorway in the Brain: A Neurologist's Search for the God Experience.* New York: Penguin, 2011.

Nord, Warren A. *Ten Essays on Good and Evil.* Chapel Hill: University of North Carolina Program in Humanities and Human Values, 2010.

Pagels, Elaine. *The Gnostic Gospels.* New York: Vintage Books, 1979.

Peake, Anthony. *The Out-of-Body Experience: The History and Science of Astral Travel.* London: Watkins, 2011.

Penrose, Roger. *Cycles of Time: An Extraordinary New View of the Universe.* New York: Alfred A. Knopf, 2010.

———. *The Emperor's New Mind.* Oxford: Oxford University Press, 1989.

———. *The Road to Reality: A Complete Guide to the Laws of the Universe.* New York: Vintage Books, 2007.

———. *Shadows of the Mind.* Oxford: Oxford University Press, 1994.

Penrose, Roger, Malcolm Longair, Abner Shimony, Nancy Cartwright, and Stephen Hawking. *The Large, The Small, and the Human Mind.* Cambridge: Cambridge University Press, 1997.

Piper, Don, and Cecil Murphey. *90 Minutes in Heaven: A True Story of Life and Death.* Grand Rapids, MI: Revell, 2004.

Reintjes, Susan. *Third Eye Open—Unmasking Your True Awareness.* Carrboro, NC: Third Eye Press, 2003.

Ring, Kenneth, and Sharon Cooper. *Mindsight: Near-Death and Out-of-Body Experiences in the Blind.* Palo Alto, CA: William James Center for Consciousness Studies at the Institute of Transpersonal Psychology, 1999.

Ring, Kenneth, and Evelyn Elsaesser Valarino. *Lessons from the Light: What We Can Learn from the Near-Death Experience.* New York: Insight Books, 1998.

Rosenblum, Bruce, and Fred Kuttner. *Quantum Enigma: Physics Encounters Consciousness.* New York: Oxford University Press, 2006.

Schroeder, Gerald L. *The Hidden Face of God: How Science Reveals the Ultimate Truth.* New York: Simon & Schuster, 2001.

Schwartz, Robert. *Your Soul's Plan: Discovering the Real Meaning of the Life You Planned Before You Were Born.* Berkeley, CA: Frog Books, 2007.

Smolin, Lee. *The Trouble with Physics.* New York. Houghton Mifflin, 2006.

Stevenson, Ian. *Children Who Remember Previous Lives: A Question of Reincarnation.* Rev. ed. Jefferson, NC: McFarland, 2001.

Sussman, Janet Iris. *The Reality of Time.* Fairfield, IA: Time Portal, 2005.

———. *Timeshift: The Experience of Dimensional Change.* Fairfield, IA: Time Portal, 1996.

Swanson, Claude. *Life Force, the Scientific Basis: Volume Two of the Synchronized Universe.* Tucson, AZ: Poseidia Press, 2010.

———. *The Synchronized Universe: New Science of the Paranormal.* Tucson, AZ: Poseidia Press, 2003.

Talbot, Michael. *The Holographic Universe.* New York: HarperCollins, 1991.

Tart, Charles T. *The End of Materialism: How Evidence of the Paranormal Is Bringing Science and Spirit Together.* Oakland, CA: New Harbinger, 2009.

Taylor, Jill Bolte. *My Stroke of Insight: A Brain Scientist's Personal Journey.* New York: Penguin, 2006.

Tipler, Frank J. *The Physics of Immortality.* New York: Doubleday, 1996.

Tompkins, Ptolemy. *The Modern Book of the Dead: A Revolutionary Perspective on Death, the Soul, and What Really Happens in the Life to Come.* New York: Atria Books, 2012.

Tononi, G. "An information integration theory of consciousness." *BMC Neuroscience* 5 (2004): 42–72.

Tucker, J. B. *Life Before Life: A Scientific Investigation of Children's Memories of Previous Lives*. New York: St. Martin's, 2005.

Tyrrell, G. N. M. *Man the Maker: A Study of Man's Mental Evolution*. New York: Dutton, 1952.

Van Lommel, Pim. *Consciousness Beyond Life: The Science of Near-Death Experience*. New York: HarperCollins, 2010.

Waggoner, Robert. *Lucid Dreaming: Gateway to the Inner Self.* Needham, MA: Moment Point Press, 2008.

Wegner, D. M. *The Illusion of Conscious Will*. Cambridge, MA: MIT Press, 2002.

Weiss, Brian L. *Many Lives, Many Masters*. New York: Fireside, 1988.

Whiteman, J. H. M. *The Mystical Life: An Outline of Its Nature and Teachings from the Evidence of Direct Experience*. London: Faber & Faber, 1961.

———. *Old & New Evidence on the Meaning of Life: The Mystical World-View and Inner Contest*. Vol. 1, *An Introduction to Scientific Mysticism*. Buckinghamshire: Colin Smythe, 1986.

Wigner, Eugene. "The Unreasonable Effectiveness of Mathematics in the Natural Sciences." *Communications in Pure and Applied Mathematics* 13, no. 1 (1960).

Wilber, Ken., ed. *Quantum Questions*. Boston: Shambhala, 1984.

Williamson, Marianne. *A Return to Love: Reflections on the Principles of a Course in Miracles*. New York: HarperCollins, 1992.

Ziewe, Jurgen. *Multidimensional Man*. Self-published, 2008.

Zukav, Gary. *The Dancing Wu Li Masters: An Overview of the New Physics*. New York: William Morrow, 1979.

Appendix A

Statement by Scott Wade, M.D.

As an infectious diseases specialist I was asked to see Dr. Eben Alexander when he presented to the hospital on November 10, 2008, and was found to have bacterial meningitis. Dr. Alexander had become ill quickly with flu-like symptoms, back pain, and a headache. He was promptly transported to the Emergency Room, where he had a CT scan of his head and then a lumbar puncture with spinal fluid suggesting a gram-negative meningitis. He was immediately begun on intravenous antibiotics targeting that and placed on a ventilator machine because of his critical condition and coma. Within twenty-four hours the gram-negative bacteria in the spinal fluid was confirmed as *E.coli*. An infection more common in infants, *E. coli* meningitis is very rare in adults (less than one in 10 million annual incidence in the United States), especially in the absence of any head trauma, neurosurgery, or other medical conditions such as diabetes. Dr. Alexander was very healthy at the time of his diagnosis and no underlying cause for his meningitis could be identified.

The mortality rate for gram-negative meningitis in children and adults ranges from 40 to 80 percent. Dr. Alexander presented to the hospital with seizures and a markedly altered mental status, both of which are risk factors for neurological complications or death (mortality over 90 percent). Despite prompt and aggressive antibiotic treatment for his *E.coli* meningitis as well as continued care in the medical intensive care unit, he remained in a coma six days and hope for a quick recovery faded (mortality over 97 percent). Then, on the seventh day, the miraculous happened—he opened his eyes, became alert, and was quickly weaned from the ventilator. The fact that he went on to have a full recovery from this illness after being in a coma for nearly a week is truly remarkable.

—Scott Wade, M.D.

Neuroscientific Hypotheses I Considered
to Explain My Experience

In reviewing my recollections with several other neurosurgeons
and scientists, I entertained several hypotheses that might explain my memories. Cutting right to the chase, they all failed
to explain the rich, robust, intricate interactivity of the Gateway
and Core experiences (the "ultra-reality"). These included:

1. A primitive brainstem program to ease terminal pain and
   suffering ("evolutionary argument" possibly as a remnant
   of "feigned-death" strategies from lower mammals?). This
   did not explain the robust, richly interactive nature of the
   recollections.

2. The distorted recall of memories from deeper parts of the
   limbic system (for example, the lateral amygdala) that have
   enough overlying brain to be relatively protected from the
   meningitic inflammation, which occurs mainly at the brain's
   surface. This did not explain the robust, richly interactive
   nature of the recollections.

3. Endogenous glutamate blockade with excitotoxicity, mim-
   icking the hallucinatory anesthetic, ketamine (occasionally
   used to explain NDEs in general). I occasionally saw the
   effects of ketamine used as an anesthetic during the earlier

part of my neurosurgical career at Harvard Medical School. The hallucinatory state it induced was most chaotic and unpleasant, and bore no resemblance whatsoever to my experience in coma.

4. N,N-dimethyltryptamine (DMT) "dump" (from the pineal, or elsewhere in the brain). DMT, a naturally occurring serotonin agonist (specifically at the 5-HT1A, 5-HT2A and 5-HT2C receptors), causes vivid hallucinations and a dreamlike state. I am personally familiar with drug experiences related to serotonin agonist/antagonists (that is, LSD, mescaline) from my teen years in the early 1970s. I have had no personal experience with DMT but have seen patients under its influence. The rich ultra-reality would still require fairly intact auditory and visual neocortex as target regions in which to generate such a rich audiovisual experience as I had in coma. Prolonged coma due to bacterial meningitis had badly damaged my neocortex, which is where all of that serotonin from the raphe nuclei in the brainstem (or DMT, a serotonin agonist) would have had effects on visual/auditory experience. But my cortex was off, and the DMT would have had no place in the brain to act. The DMT hypothesis failed on the basis of the ultra-reality of the audiovisual experience, and lack of cortex on which to act.

5. Isolated preservation of cortical regions might have explained some of my experience, but were most unlikely, given the severity of my meningitis and its refractoriness to therapy for a week: peripheral white blood cell (WBC) count over 27,000 per mm^3, 31 percent bands with toxic granulations, CSF WBC count over 4,300 per mm^3, CSF

glucose down to 1.0 mg/dl, CSF protein 1,340 mg/dl, diffuse meningeal involvement with associated brain abnormalities revealed on my enhanced CT scan, and neurological exams showing severe alterations in cortical function and dysfunction of extraocular motility, indicative of brainstem damage.

6. In an effort to explain the "ultra-reality" of the experience, I examined this hypothesis: Was it possible that networks of inhibitory neurons might have been predominantly affected, allowing for unusually high levels of activity among the excitatory neuronal networks to generate the apparent "ultra-reality" of my experience? One would expect meningitis to preferentially disturb the superficial cortex, possibly leaving deeper layers partially functional. The computing unit of the neocortex is the six-layered "functional column," each with a lateral diameter of 0.2–0.3 mm. There is significant interwiring laterally to immediately adjacent columns in response to modulatory control signals that originate largely from subcortical regions (the thalamus, basal ganglia, and brainstem). Each functional column has a component at the surface (layers 1–3), so that meningitis effectively disrupts the function of each column just by damaging the surface layers of the cortex. The anatomical distribution of inhibitory and excitatory cells, which have a fairly balanced distribution within the six layers, does not support this hypothesis. Diffuse meningitis over the brain's surface effectively disables the entire neocortex due to this columnar architecture. Full-thickness destruction is unnecessary for total functional disruption. Given the prolonged course of my poor neurological function (seven days) and the severity

of my infection, it is unlikely that even deeper layers of the cortex were still functioning.

7. The thalamus, basal ganglia, and brainstem are deeper brain structures ("subcortical regions") that some colleagues postulated might have contributed to the processing of such hyperreal experiences. In fact, none of those structures could play any such role without having at least some regions of the neocortex still intact. All agreed in the end that such subcortical structures alone could not have handled the intense neural calculations required for such a richly interactive experiential tapestry.

8. A "reboot phenomenon"—a random dump of bizarre disjointed memories due to old memories in the damaged neocortex, which might occur on restarting the cortex into consciousness after a prolonged system-wide failure, as in my diffuse meningitis. Especially given the intricacies of my elaborate recollections, this seems most unlikely.

9. Unusual memory generation through an archaic visual pathway through the midbrain, prominently used in birds but only rarely identifiable in humans. It can be demonstrated in humans who are cortically blind, due to damaged occipital cortex. It provided no clue as to the ultra-reality I witnessed, and failed to explain the auditory-visual interleaving.

Index

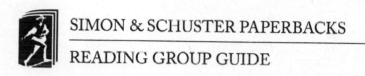

SIMON & SCHUSTER PAPERBACKS
READING GROUP GUIDE

PROOF

of

HEAVEN

Introduction

As a neurosurgeon schooled in some of the most elite institutions of the American scientific community, Dr. Eben Alexander considered himself an "unbeliever"—one who did not believe in God, Heaven or an afterlife. He was confident that the brain was the ultimate source of consciousness and all reports of experiences in the "spiritual realm" were unsupportable from a scientific perspective. Everything changed, though, on November 10, 2008, when a splitting headache landed him in an emergency room and ultimately a seven-day coma. In *Proof of Heaven*, Dr. Alexander recounts the story of those seven days and the spiritually transforming experience that occurred during them. When he awakened from his coma, his old certainties about the nonexistence of the afterlife were gone.

Topics & Questions for Discussion

1. Do you know anyone who had a Near Death Experience (NDE)? What was your attitude toward their experience when they described it to you?

2. How does the fact that the author (Eben Alexander) is a physician (neurosurgeon) influence your attitude toward his story of his NDE?

3. In chapter 10, "What Counts," the author shares some of his family history and how, after learning some news about his birth parents as an adult, he lost his "last, half-acknowledged hope that there was some personal element in the universe . . ." Do you identify with that hope? Has there been a time in your life when that hope was either confirmed or lost?

4. On pp. 57–58, the author poses these questions: "Was there a force or intelligence watching out for all of us? Who cared about humans in a truly loving way?" How would you answer those questions? How have you come to those answers?

5. In chapter 11, "An End to the Downward Spiral," the author describes the impact of meeting his birth family and learning about aspects of his life story that he had not previously known about. Why do you think these experiences had such a significant impact on his sense of well-being? Have you ever had an experience in which you learned new things about your own life story? How did your experience change you?

6. On page 71, the author puts into words the wordless message he received during his NDE. "You are loved and cherished. You have nothing to fear. There is nothing you can do wrong." How does this message make you feel? What emotions do you experience when you read the words? Do you believe they are true?

7. On page 73, the author asserts that ". . . certain members of the scientific community, who are pledged to the materialist worldview, have insisted again and again that science and spirituality cannot coexist." What is the materialist worldview? Do you believe science and spirituality are necessarily opposed? Describe.

8. On page 76, the author states: "The (false) suspicion that we can somehow be separated from God is the root of every form of anxiety in the universe . . ." Do you agree? Why or why not?

9. In chapter 14, the author describes one factor that made his NDE unique. What was this factor? Do you agree with the author that it really does set his experience apart?

10. How does the author's response to his NDE make you feel about your own faith? Do you agree with his conclusion on page 96: "None of us are ever unloved. Each and every one of us is deeply known and cared for by a Creator who cherishes us beyond any ability we have to comprehend"? How do his conclusions compare and contrast with your understanding of God?

11. What part of Dr. Alexander's story moved you the most? Describe.

12. Upon his first visit to his Episcopal church after "returning" to his body, Dr. Alexander said: "At last, I understood what religion was really all about. Or at least was supposed to be about. I didn't just believe in God; I knew God" (p. 148). What do you think is the difference between believing in God and knowing God?

13. In chapter 31, the author describes three varieties of attitude toward NDEs. With which do you most identify? Has reading this book moved you from one group to another?

14 On page 141, the author makes the bold statement that scientists in our society are "the official gatekeepers on the matter of what's real and what isn't." Do you think this is true? If it is, why do you think scientists have been given this kind of authority? Do you think this authority really should belong to scientists? Why or why not?

15. On page 103, the author describes the positive effect his friends' prayers had during his coma. Does this part of his story resonate with you? Do you have any experience(s) of your own of prayers being effective?

16. How do you feel about the title of the book? Do you think spiritual experiences and realities can be proven? In what ways does the author's suggestion that a spiritual experience can be proven help or hinder his story's believability?

Enhance Your Book Club

1. If you know someone who has experienced an NDE, invite them to your next book club meeting and ask them to share their story. How comfortable or uncomfortable is the group with the sense of mystery and the unknown? How do different members of the group respond to things that are beyond our ability to fully comprehend?

2. Keep a month-long log of things you notice in your life that can't be reduced to material or physical explanations (i.e., anything that happens that has an element of mystery or transcendence). Bring your log to your next book club and discuss the options for how to think about these realities.

3. Read *The Universe Next Door: A Basic Worldview Catalog*, which provides an overview of the eight main worldviews that are held by different individuals in the twentieth century. At your next book club meeting, discuss which worldview you most identify with and why.

4. Think about the power of science in affecting your own beliefs. Are you a person of faith, science, or both? Discuss.

A Conversation with Eben Alexander, M.D.

1. Why did you decide to become a physician and specifically a neurosurgeon?

My father certainly had a lot to do with it. As I describe in the book, he was a celebrated neurosurgeon who had a huge influence not just on me, but on just about everyone he met. That would have been about the end of it if you'd asked me this question before my NDE. Now it's a little different. I see my father's role in my life as part of what you might call my destiny. I think my life this time around was supposed to be about delving into the mystery of consciousness and how it relates to our fundamental understanding of reality.

2. How has your NDE changed the way you make decisions about how to spend your time and energy each day and the way you relate to others?

I was never much of a time waster. Even when "relaxing" I was usually going in overdrive. That's even more the case now. I see time as more precious than ever. But at the same time, if something goes wrong, I'm able to take it much more in stride. Every moment of our life is precious beyond measure. But it's not all we have. There is more—much more—to come.

In terms of relationships with others, everything has changed. I see all those around me as eternal spiritual beings undergoing the glories and trials of the physical world. This does not mean I'm wearing rose-colored glasses, however. Hardship and suffering appear in a clearer focus and in fact hit me harder than they did before. Seeing the world more deeply does not mean filtering the negative out. It just means seeing it in its true context.

3. Has your NDE impacted the way you practice medicine and/or interact with your patients?

My current schedule has become far too busy with presentations and telling my story to leave time for patient care. I hope to get back to it at some point, but with a different focus. I plan on working with patients who are terminal, in ICU or hospice, and in helping families deal with the impending loss of a loved one. I have so much more to offer them now. I feel that that is one of the main reasons I returned—to share my story and give real comfort to those who need it most.

4. In the earlier part of your book, you talk about your hope for what you describe as a "personal element in the universe" (p. 57). That hope seems to have been realized in the encounter with a personal Creator that you describe occurring during your NDE (p. 96). Yet you also state that "*consciousness is the basis of all that exists*" (p. 154), and this has a less personal sound to it. Can you elaborate on this contrast?

Consciousness is a primary aspect of the universe and a supreme mystery that transcends all our efforts to capture it. But that doesn't mean we shouldn't try to describe it anyhow, and in doing so we can go more in one direction or another. That is, we can zero in on its less personal aspects or its more personal ones. But the loving Creator I encountered was very definitely *not* impersonal. At the same time, calling that Creator "personal" is problematic too, because it introduces limitations. The same kind of limitations that are introduced when we use words like "Him" or "Her" or "It" to describe that Creator. The reality of the Divine burns all these terms instantly to ash.

5. The word "Proof" in the title has caused controversy. Do you think using this word has helped or hindered you in your efforts to demonstrate the reality of the spiritual world?

I wanted it known that this was not just another NDE story. My experience provides extremely strong evidence that consciousness is not dependent on the cortex. It was proof for me personally, and it has convinced many others. The cortex mediates consciousness while we are on earth, it does not produce it. Of that I am certain. So while I completely understand the difficulties that people have had with the title, in the end I feel it is accurate.

6. In chapter 32 of the book, you briefly allude to going to church after you recovered an understanding of "what religion was really all about. Or at least was supposed to be about." Can you say more about what you realized at that moment?

I felt deeply, for the first time in a place of worship, the concrete presence of the Divine. The images and symbols around me struck me with a power that I had never appreciated before. I have since visited many places of worship, both Christian and otherwise, and though the specifics of the settings differ, that core feeling of gratitude to the Divine always comes through.

7. As a young man you thought science had all the answers. How would you advise a current medical student to approach the argument (popular among scientists) that we are "fast approaching a Theory of Everything (or TOE),

which would not seem to leave much room for our soul, or spirit, or for Heaven, and God"? (pp. 153–54).

It's easy to be fooled into thinking that you know all there is to know. The history of science and philosophy is filled with examples of thinkers who were tempted into believing they could do just that. When I was in med school, the thinking was very much: *we don't know everything about the universe yet, but we're just about to.* I now find that idea absolutely laughable in its arrogance and its blindness. We don't have the first hint about how the universe really works or what's really in it. We have no idea what dark matter is, we have no idea what consciousness is. We have no idea how many dimensions there are to the universe, how populated or unpopulated they are by other consciousnesses. One could go on. I would advise someone in medical school now to thank their stars they are living in a time when we do know so much about the universe, about the human body, about all manner of things that we were essentially in the dark about just a hundred years ago. But there's a big difference between feeling grateful about the knowledge we do have and thinking we know everything. We don't, and never will.

8. Are you still in touch with your birth family?

Yes I am. My birth family and my adoptive family have become very close, and we have all grown in many wonderful ways as a result of our reunion.

9. What was the most challenging part of writing your story?

The most challenging part was simply containing my sheer excitement and enthusiasm to tell the world what had happened to me. What I experienced was not new. Many others have caught a glimpse of the realms I encountered during my NDE and told of them. But the medical facts behind my case *were* new, and once the full force of this came home to me, it was very hard to keep patient during the long process of creating the book. The early drafts read more like a telegram than a book. I gave all the details of what happened to me within the first few pages, because I was just so anxious to tell the reader how amazing it all was. Learning to slow down and do it right was hard. The final manuscript of *Proof of Heaven* was produced with the help of a friend of mine, a gifted writer named Ptolemy Tompkins, who had written a book, *The Modern Book of the Dead*, with which I'd identified closely. Along with my editor, Priscilla Painton, Ptolemy showed me that one of the most extraordinary things about my story is that it is just that: *a story*. It needed to unfold piece by piece and revelation by revelation, just as it did in real life.

10. How has this experience changed your life?

It has changed everything imaginable in my life. However, I continue to struggle through life's bumps and surprises like everyone else. Like many people who have undergone a spiritually transformative experience of such magnitude, I have no choice but to live my life as authentically as I can. We must always be true to our hearts.

11. What is the main thing you hope people take away from reading your story?

That we are *far more* than physical beings. Not only do we continue to exist after bodily death, but our awareness functions at a much higher level once it is free from the physical limitations of the brain. At the core of our existence is a love for us far grander than we can ever imagine: the infinite, unconditional love of a Divine Creator. That love offers us the power to heal ourselves, our species, our planet and our entire existence.

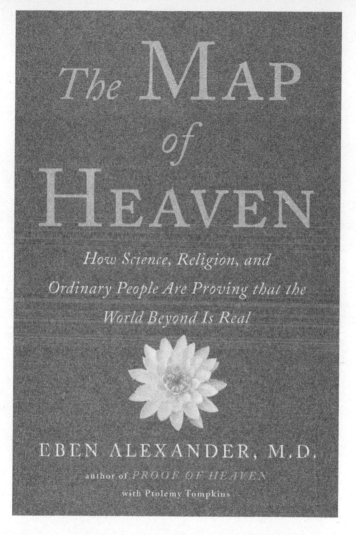